Mrs J Shillito
47 Dean Park Drive
Drighlington
BRADFORD
BD11 1AL

CW01597334

FATS & FIGURES

by **Karen Daly**

About the Author

Karen Daly

A former Mrs. Australia and 4th runner up Mrs. World, Karen Daly pursues an active career as a model with Vivien's, one of Australia's leading agencies.

Originally a N.S.W. representative swimmer and N.S.W.A.S.A. swim instructor, Karen has worked in the health, fitness and beauty industry for many years, currently combining her work as a qualified A.F.A.C. fitness instructor, supervisor and personal trainer with her career in the modelling industry.

Karen is married to noted jazz musician and big band Maestro Warren Daly.

Thank You

WARREN

Not only for your faith in me, but also for your unending patience, support and assistance.

ACKNOWLEDGEMENTS

The author would like to acknowledge the following sources of reference and thank those companies who so kindly shared their information:-

A.A.Tegel Pty. Limited
Aminoactive Australia
Ardmona Foods Limited
Arnott's Biscuits Limited
Arriba Burritos (Pattie's Bakery Pty.Ltd.)
Associated Baking Corporation
Attiki Pty.Ltd.
Aussie Bodies
Australasian Soft Drink Association Ltd.
Australian Co-Operative Foods Limited
Australian Dairy Corporation
Australian Dried Fruits Sales Pty.Ltd.
Australian Meat & Livestock Corporation
Australian Pork Corporation
Australian Quality Egg Farms Ltd.
Australian United Foods (Qld.)
Baitz Liquors (Inchcape Liquor Marketing)
Baskin Robbins (Graham Services Pty.Ltd.)
Bellis Fruit Bars
Berrima Cookie Co.
Berrivale Orchards Limited
Bonlac Foods Limited
Bradsnax Foods Pty.Ltd.
Bronte Industries Pty.Ltd.
Brunswick (Grocery Corporation Pty.Ltd.)
Bulla (Regal Cream Products Pty.Ltd.)
Cadbury Schweppes Pty.Ltd.
C & M Antoniou Pty.Ltd.
Campbell's Soups Australia
Canned Food Information Service Inc.
Cantarella Bros.Pty Ltd.(Norwegian Dairies)
C.C.A. Beverages
Cerebos (Australia) Limited
Charioto Products
C.H.Chang Distributors
Chisholm Manufacturing
Chris' Greek Dips
Clarke's Cookie Company
(Auto-Bake Pty Ltd)
Confectionery Manufacturers of
Australasia
Consolidated Biscuits Pty Ltd
Creative Gourmet Pty.Limited.
Dairy Bell (Ice Cream(Aust)Pty Ltd)
Darrell Lea Chocolate Shops Pty.Ltd.
Defiance Quality Foods
Dollars Sweets Company
(Aust.) Pty. Ltd.
Edgell-Birds Eye
Erica Specialties
Farmland (Coles Supermarkets
Aust. Pty.Ltd.)
Ferrero Australia Pty.Ltd.
Findus Frozen Foods
Fish Marketing Authority
F. Mayer Imports Pty. Ltd.
Food Technology in Australia Vol39(5)
Franklins Limited
George Weston Foods Limited
Gisé Crème Glacé
Glenny's (Glenn Foods, Inc.)
Go 4 It Fast Foods Pty.Ltd.
Golden Circle Limited
Gold Medal Snacks Pty.Ltd.
Go Natural Australia
Goodman Fielder Limited
Green's General Foods Pty.Limited
Griffins Foods Limited
Griffs Prepared Foods
Hans Continental Smallgoods Pty.Ltd.
Health Minders Pty.Limited
Heather Brae Shortbreads Pty.Ltd.
Henry Jones Foods (IXL)
Herbert Adams Bakeries
H.J.Heinz Company Australia Ltd.

ACKNOWLEDGEMENTS

House of Treats
Hungry Jack's Pty.Ltd.
I & J Foods Limited
In Foods (Meloats Health Bars)
Inghams Enterprises Pty.Linited
Jacobs Suchard(Australia) Pty.Ltd.
Jalna Dairy Foods Pty.Ltd.
K & S Indian Foods
Kellogg (Aust.)Pty.Ltd.
K.F.C.
Kitchens of Sara Lee(Australia)Pty.Ltd.
Kiwi Brands Pty.Ltd.
K.L.Valentine Pty.Ltd.
Kraft Foods Limited
Lactos Pty.Ltd.
Lanes Biscuits Pty.Ltd.
Latina Pasta House
Le Traiteur Pty.Ltd.
Limmits Biscuits
Logan Farm Pty.Ltd.
Longa Life Vegetarian Products Pty.Ltd.
Lowan Whole Foods Pty.Ltd.
Magic Apple
Mainland Dairies Pty.Ltd.
Malibu(Twelve Islands Shipping Co.Limited)
Makmur Enterprises Pty.Ltd.
Margaret's Kitchen Australia Pty.Ltd.
Mars Confectionery of Australia
Master Foods of Australia
McCain Foods (Aust.)Pty.Ltd.
McCormick Foods Australia Pty.Ltd.
McDonald's Australia Limited
Meadow Lea Foods Limited
Mellow Yellow Products Pty.Limited
Menora Gourmet Products Pty.Ltd (Danish Luxury Cakes, Jacob's Biscuits)
Milk Marketing(NSW) Pty. Limited
Mother Earth Fine Foods Pty.Ltd.
Mums Food Distribution (Pasta di Casa)
Murray Goulburn Co-Operative Limited
Musashi Pty.Ltd.
Nana Diver's Pty.Ltd.
National Dairies Ltd.
National Pies Pty.Ltd.
Naturally Good Products Pty.Ltd.
Naytura Cookies (Safeway, a division of Woolworths Limited)
Nestlé Australia Ltd.
Nestlé Confectionery Ltd.
Nicherei Australia Pty.Ltd.
Norco Co-Operative Limited
Nutritional Values of Australian Foods, (National Food Authority)
Orchy Fruit Juices
Orgran Natural Food Products
Pacific Beverages Australia Pty.Ltd.
Pacific Food Products (Australasia) Pty. Ltd.
Pampas (a Div. of Quality Bakers Aust. Ltd)
Paradise Food Industries Pty.Ltd.
Paramount Seafood (Grocery Corp. Pty.Ltd.)
Pasta House Mfg. Co. Pty. Ltd.
Peck's Australia Pty. Limited
Pepsi-Cola Bottlers Australia
Peters & Brownes Group
Peters Foods
Pizza Hut Australia
Players Biscuits Pty. Ltd.
Poseidon Tarama Pty. Ltd.
Powerbar
Pryde's Sweets Pty. Ltd.
Pure & Natural Juices Pty. Ltd.
Quality Bakers Australia Limited
Queensco-Unity Dairy Foods Co-Op. Ass. Ltd.
Q.U.F. Industries Ltd.

ACKNOWLEDGEMENTS

R & C Products Pty. Ltd (Reckitt & Colman)
Red Rooster Foods
Ricegrowers' Co-Operative Limited
Riviana Foods Pty.Ltd.
Ronnoco Foods Pty.Ltd.
Safcol Australia Pty.Ltd.
Sanitarium Health Food Company
San Remo Macaroni Company Pty.Ltd.
Sargents Pty.Ltd.
Schweppes Cottees
Sealord Products Limited
Socomin International Fine Foods (Bahlsen, Droste, Fazer Chocolates, McVitie's)
Southern Country Foods Pty. Ltd.
S.P.C. Limited
Spring Valley Beverages Pty.Ltd.
Steggles Foods (a Division of Australian Poultry Limited)
Streets Ice Cream Pty. Limited
Stuart Alexander & Co. Pty. Ltd. (Anthon Berg, Betty Crocker, Lindt, Mentos,Paynes)
Sunburst Regency Foods Pty. Limited
Sun Health Foods
Sunrise Confectioners(Aust.) Pty. Ltd.
Sunvalley Australia Pty.Ltd.
Superpop Pty. Ltd.
Susan Day Cakes Pty. Ltd.
Sydney Popcorn Co Pty. Ltd.
Tamarama Fresh Juices Australia Pty. Ltd.
Tastee Products
The Aeroplane Jelly Company
The Australian Dairy Corporation
The Australian Nutrition Foundation Inc.
The Bega Co-Operative Society Ltd
The French Kitchen
The Healthy Snak People
The Phoenix Biscuit Co.
The Smith's Snackfood Company Ltd.
The Sunraysia Natural Beverage Co. Pty. Ltd.
The Uncle Tobys Company Pty .Ltd.
The Vege Chip Company Pty. Ltd.
The Webster Biscuit Co.
Tip Top Bakeries - National
Tixana Pty. Ltd.
Très Bon Continental Bakeries
Unibic
Unifoods
United Dairies Pty. Ltd.
United Distillers (Aust.) Limited
Valcorp Holdings Pty. Ltd. (Casa Fiesta)
Wander (Australia) Pty. Ltd.
Weis Frozen Foods
West Coast Cooler (Southcorp Wines Pty. Ltd)
Willow Valley Products Pty. Limited
World's Finest Chocolate Australia Pty. Ltd.
Wendys New South Wales (Oraka Pty. Ltd)
Yoplait Australia
Z & E Health Bars Pty. Ltd.

First Published November, 1994

by ROCK WALLABY ENTERPRISES PTY. LTD.
ACN 066 852 042
Level 2, 454-456 Pacific Highway,
St. Leonards NSW 2065
Enquiries: Contact FATS AND FIGURES: 042 265 490

Printed by McPherson's Printing Group, Sydney

Re-printed by McPherson's Printing Group, MAY 1995

2nd Re-print by McPherson's Printing Group, SEPTEMBER 1995

3rd Re-print by McPherson's Printing Group, MAY 1996

Typeset by QuoArt Pty. Ltd., Wollongong

Cover Photography by Suzie Mitchell, Twenty Two Pty. Ltd., Sydney

Copyright © Rock Wallaby Enterprises Pty. Ltd. 1994

All rights reserved. No part of this publication may be reproduced, stored in a retrieval system, or transmitted in any form or by any means, electronic, mechanical, photocopying, recording or otherwise, without the prior written permission of the publisher.

This book is for PRIVATE USE ONLY. LOAN OR HIRE of the book or any part is NOT PERMITTED.

ISBN 0 646 21528 0

This book is published for the consumer's convenience as an easy reference guide only. It is not intended as a substitute for personalised consultation with your doctor.

The author and publisher of this book are not medically trained and are not licensed to give medical advice. Always consult with your doctor before embarking on any dietary course.

The fat and calorie figures provided are based on the author's extensive research conducted throughout 1994 however the contents of products are subject to change by manufacturers from time to time and those contents may currently vary from those listed in this book.

Information in this book is not an endorsement or recommendation of any product, manufacturers, companies or individuals.

The author and publisher each disclaim any liability, damage or loss whatsoever arising directly or indirectly from this book, the information contained in it or its use.

CONTENTS

Page

Introduction 1
- Fats Vs Calories 2
- Not all Calories are Equal 2
- Why Eat Less Fat? 3
- Fat - How Much? 4
- Your Own Personal 'Fat Budget' 7
- How to Add up your 'Fat Budget' Score 7
- No Hunger Pangs - Eat What You Like 8
- Exercise Connection 8
- Tips on Avoiding Fat Filled Foods 10
- Abbreviations 12
- How to Use 'Fats & Figures' 12

Fats & Figures.......

Alcohol, see Drinks Alcoholic 78
Biscuits, Crackers, Crispbreads 13
Breads, Bread Rolls, Crumpets, Bagels, Muffins, Croissants 27
- Breadcrumbs, Bread Mixes, Breadsticks
- Crumpets & Muffins
- Pita Breads, Pizza Bases

Breakfast Cereals 33
Cakes & Desserts - Fresh 38
- Muffins
- Karen's fat free Muffin Recipe
- Desserts - fresh
- Crepes, Pancakes, Pikelets, Waffles
- Dairy Desserts
- Packet, Fresh, Frozen & Canned
- Jellies

Cheese & Cheese Products 56
- Cheese Sauce
- Cheese Spreads
- Cheese/Dairy Dips
- Cottage Cheese
- Cream & Fruit Cheese
- Processed Cheese
- Ricotta Cheese

Chocolate & Confectionery 61
- Boxed Chocolates
- Chocolate Coated Fruit & Nuts
- Easter Eggs

CONTENTS

Page

Cooking - Baking Products 75
Arrowroot, Cornflour
Baking Powder, Baking Soda, Bicarb Soda
Cake Decorations, Frosting, Marzipan
Carob Powder, Carob Bits, Cooking Chocolate
Cocoa Powder, Coconut, Custard Powder
Essences, Gelatine
Mixed Peel, Fruit Mince
Poppy, Sesame, Sunflower Seeds
Yeast, Whey
Dips, Dip Mixes, Salsa Dips 77
Diet Shakes - see Protein Powders & Meal Replacers 173
Drinks - Alcoholic 78
Drinks - Non-alcoholic 82
Bovril, Bonox
Chocolate
Coffee, fresh, packaged mixes, liquer
Coffee substitutes
Cordial, Rosehip syrup
Milkshakes, Thickshakes
Mineral Water, Still, Sparkling, Flavoured
Powdered Drinks (Milo, Quik etc.)
Soft Drinks
Sports - Athelic Drinks, powders
Tea
Eggs, Egg Drinks, Egg Meals 86
Fats, Butter, Margarine 88
Cream
Oils
Sour Cream
Fish - Fresh, Frozen 90
Fish Meals
Shellfish
Canned Fish, Fish Spreads
Flours & Grains 98
Fruit - Fresh 99
Crystallised, Dried, Frozen, Glacé
Canned
Snacks
Fruit Juices 106
Game - see Meats 156
Gravy - see Stock & Flavourings 212

CONTENTS

Page

Health Bars & Confectionery 112
Health Snack Foods & Muesli Bars 116
Herbs & Spices - see Stock & Flavourings 212
Ice Cream & Ice Confections 121
Frozen Yoghurt
Ice Cream Cones
Ice Cream Toppings
Jam - see Sandwich Spreads 188
Jelly - see Cakes & Desserts 55
Legumes & Beans - see Vegetables 228
Meal Replacers - see Protein Powders 173
Meals - Pies 130
Frozen, Packet & Canned
Vegetarian
Meat - Beef 149
Beef Mince
Lamb
Pork
Bacon & Ham
Veal
Sausages
Rabbit
Game
Gourmet & Specialty
Offal
Smallgoods, Processed, Cold & Continental Meats
Milk 163
Condensed
Evaporated
Flavoured Milk Drinks
Longlife
Powdered
Soy, Various Other Milks
Muesli Bars - see Health Snack Foods 116
Nuts & Seeds - Fresh, Packet 167
Nut & Seed Pastes, Spreads
Pasta, Spaghetti, Noodles 169
Pastry - Fresh, Frozen 171
Pizza - Frozen, (also see Take Away Foods) 172
Karen's Low Fat Pizza Recipe

CONTENTS

Page

Poultry 159
- Chicken
- Chicken Smallgoods
- Duck, Goose, Hare
- Turkey, Turkey Smallgoods

Protein Powders, Diet Shakes & Meal Replacers 173
Restaurants - Ethnic Cuisine 175
- Asian
- Greek
- Indian
- Italian
- Lebanese
- Mexican & Spanish

Rice 182
- Rice Bran
- Rice Cakes
- Rice Dishes

Salads - Fresh, Tinned 183
Salad Dressings 184
Sandwiches 186
Sandwich Spreads - Toast Toppers 188
- Cheese, Chocolate, Fruit, Nut Spreads
- Fish & Meat Pastes
- Honey, Syrup
- Jam
- Paté
- Peanut Butter, Lemon Butter
- Vegemite

Sauces & Condiments 190
- Olives
- Pickles, Relishes
- Salsa
- Tomato Paste, Purée

Seeds - see Nuts 167
Snack Foods -Potato Crisps, Popcorn, Pretzels 200
- Cheese Snacks
- Corn Chips
- Fruit & Nut Mixes
- Nibble Mixes
- Rice Crackers

CONTENTS

Page

Soups - Packet & Canned 204
Soybean Foods - see Vegetables 230
Stock & Flavourings 212
- Gravy
- Herbs & Spices

Sugar & Sweeteners 213
- Honey
- Syrups
- Toppings

Take Away & Fast Foods 214
- Chinese, Asian, Greek, Lebanese, Italian, Mexican
- Chicken
- Chips
- Fish
- Hamburgers
- Milkshakes
- Pies, Pasties & Sausage Rolls
- Pizza
- Quiche
- Miscellaneous (Fairy Floss, Hot Dogs, Rissoles)
- Popular Take-Away Outlets

Vegetables - Fresh, Canned, Frozen & Dried 222
- Fat Free Hot Chips
- Legumes & Beans
- Soybean Foods

Yoghurt 234
- see Ice Confections for Frozen Yoghurt
- Yoghurt Coated Confectionery, see Health Bars & Confectionery

INTRODUCTION

This reference book began as a project for myself when I decided to limit the amount of fat in my everyday diet for general health and weight loss.

However, I found it extremely difficult to glean the information that I needed to achieve my aim, as I could find no publications that described the amount of fat in particular foodstuffs - especially my favourite brands.

So I set about the lengthy task of finding out the information that I wanted. Many months, hundreds of letters and several huge telephone bills later, when it was all compiled, I realised that many others may be just as confused as I had been and might also like to know exactly 'Where The Fat Is'.

That is when I decided to publish this book and share this enlightening information.

Like many people, I have tried a multitude of different 'diets' over the years. Whilst some of them resulted in a reasonable weight loss (mostly water, not body fat), they were all accompanied by the associated feelings of deprivation and often plain old hunger! And, inevitably, the weight soon went back on again as well.

I have worked in the modelling and fitness industries for many years and have always been interested in pursuing a healthy lifestyle and broadening my experience and knowledge whenever I was able. It was whilst working as a fitness instructor that I became increasingly interested in the 'low fat' way of eating (notice I did not say DIET!) and the theory behind it.

Not only is it possible to lose weight and keep it off, but also to enjoy a healthier, longer life by reducing the amount of fat in our everyday diet.

Research is leading us to a new concept of controlling the amount of fat we eat and not being obsessed with just counting calories. In other words, it is more important to limit our daily fat intake rather than just count the calories. By restricting the fat intake to a lower level the calorie intake will automatically be less important.

As an aerobics instructor, it is important for me to keep my energy intake (ie. my calorie intake) moderate to high to enable me to have the stamina to get through my classes and training routine - so restricting my calorie intake has always been undesirable. Now, if I wish to lose weight, I simply keep my calories to a moderate level and restrict my fat intake to 10% (until I have lost the weight I want to) AND I can choose which foods I want to eat, too.

No deprivation, no hunger pangs, no problem!

FAT vs CALORIES

When energy (calorie) intake is reduced to a very low level such as on a restrictive low calorie diet, your body's metabolism automatically slows down because it is protecting you from what it sees as an impending famine. (Your metabolism is the rate at which your body burns fuel/energy/calories - whether performing normal bodily functions such as breathing, or whether to get you through an exercise session).

When your metabolism slows down then your body burns energy/calories even slower! Hence the endless dieting yo-yo. Your body will stop you from losing fat because it is saving your fat stores for what it thinks is the onset of starvation.

So don't starve yourself of calories on fad diets. What you need to concentrate on is the amount of fat that you consume each day and that is where you should use this book as a reference until you become familiar with which foods are low in fat.

Much of the weight loss from very restrictive low calorie diets is a result of the loss of water and lean body mass (muscle) which shows up on your bathroom scales as weight loss. This in itself has a negative effect on your metabolism because when you lose muscle tissue your metabolism will slow down even further.

Muscle tissue in the body uses more energy/calories than adipose (body fat) tissue does. So the higher your muscle to body fat ratio is, the faster your metabolism will work. So, the aim when losing weight is not to lose water and muscle but to lose BODY FAT.

When you decrease the fat content in your diet to the suggested levels, you WILL lose body fat.

Remember however, that when you combine exercise (see section on Exercise Connection) with a low fat intake, you will see even better results because you will be building your lean body mass (your muscles) and losing fat body mass (fat) at the same time. Whilst aesthetically pleasing, initially this may not always show up as an immediate 'weight' loss on your bathroom scales because you will have gained some muscle mass and muscle weights more than fat.

The best way to keep track of your fat loss (without the expert help of body fat callipers or an immersion tank) is to keep a fortnightly record of your measurements. Weigh yourself once a week - not every day.

NOT ALL CALORIES ARE EQUAL

For the purposes of this book I have used the older term of calorie rather than kilojoule. If you wish to convert calories to kilojoules you simply multiply the calories by 4.2.

Each type of food that we eat has a different caloric value:-

Carbohydrates have 4 calories per gram.
Proteins have 4 calories per gram.
Alcohol has 7 calories per gram.

Fats have 9 calories per gram!!!

ie. FAT CONTAINS MORE THAN TWICE AS MANY CALORIES AS PROTEIN AND CARBOHYDRATE

Recent studies have shown that 'dieters' will achieve better and longer term results by restricting their fat intake instead of just restricting their calorie intake.

Research has also found that when we consume carbohydrates (bread, pasta, vegetables, fruit etc.), these are easily converted into energy for our bodies to use for exercise or general activities.

However, when we consume fat it is more easily stored straight into our bodies as fat (adipose tissue). It is then harder for our bodies to convert this fat into energy for us to use. So when you eat that tablespoon of butter, think of where it ends up.

When you need a sweet treat, reach for fresh or dried fruit - if these do not help, then instead of satisfying your craving with a high fat 'sweet' treat such as chocolate or biscuits, it is better to eat a fat free 'sweet' treat like jelly beans (not the whole packet). Another great low fat 'sweet' snack is the humble crumpet - forget the butter or margarine and just spread with some of your favourite jam or honey.

WHY EAT LESS FAT?

Most nutritionists and health industry workers would agree that Australians and the western world in general consume far too much fat in their everyday diet.

Many people are consuming 40-50% of their daily intake as fat. This amount of fat could weigh up to 165 grams per day - 1155 grams in one week! (One tub of margarine weighs 375 grams thus, in one week, this amount of fat consumption would equal the weight of almost 3 tubs of margarine!). Now that cannot be considered healthy.

It is widely recommended that a healthier range to aim for is 30% of our total energy (calorie) intake as fat. I believe that this figure is still too generous and have found that a lower level of 20% for general health, well being and weight maintenance is more realistic for long term benefits. Further, I believe that a level of 10-15% is the most successful and realistic for any one wishing to lose weight.

It is well documented that consuming too much fat can cause many health problems including obesity, high cholesterol and subsequent increased risks of high blood pressure and heart disease. All excellent reasons for lowering your fat consumption.

However, it is important to remember that some fat in our diet is necessary for good health. It provides us with body fat which protects the body's internal organs and it also provides vitamins such as A, D and E.

Most of us do not set out to eat so much fat - often it just creeps up on us without our realising. This reference guide can help you to keep track of how much fat you eat.

Fat measurements are given in grams and I will refer to how many grams of fat are in particular products throughout this book.

FAT - HOW MUCH?

Firstly, you will need to know what your daily calorie intake is. If you do not already know then consult the Fats & Figures TABLE "A" listed below:-

Fats & Figures: Table "A"

GUIDELINES FOR DAILY CALORIE INTAKE REQUIREMENTS

Women		Men	
Ideal Body Weight	**Calorie Intake RANGE**	**Ideal Body Weight**	**Calorie Intake RANGE**
40.0 kg	1300 - 1600	55.0 kg	1800 - 2300
42.5 kg	1350 - 1650	57.5 kg	1850 - 2350
45.0 kg	1400 - 1700	60.0 kg	1900 - 2400
47.5 kg	1450 - 1750	62.5 kg	1950 - 2470
50.0 kg	1500 - 1800	65.0 kg	2000 - 2550
52.5 kg	1525 - 1850	67.5 kg	2050 - 2630
55.0 kg	1550 - 1900	70.0 kg	2100 - 2700
57.5 kg	1575 - 1950	72.5 kg	2150 - 2770
60.0 kg	1600 - 2000	75.0 kg	2200 - 2850
62.5 kg	1625 - 2050	77.5 kg	2250 - 2930
65.0 kg	1650 - 2100	80.0 kg	2300 - 3000
67.5 kg	1675 - 2150	82.5 kg	2350 - 3070
70.0 kg	1700 - 2200	85.0 kg	2400 - 3150
72.5 kg	1725 - 2250	87.5 kg	2470 - 3230
75.0 kg	1750 - 2300	90.0 kg	2500 - 3300
77.5 kg	1800 - 2400	92.5 kg	2630 - 3400
80.0 kg	1870 - 2500	95.0 kg	2700 - 3500
		97.5 kg	2800 - 3650
		100.0 kg	2900 - 3800

Table "A" should be used as a guide only. Calorie requirements can vary from those listed depending on your age, frame, activity level etc. The figures given in Table "A" are for a person of medium frame.

When finding the calorie range applicable to your desired body weight, you need to take into consideration your physical activity level:

* If you are inactive and do not exercise at all then you should use the lower figure in your calorie intake range.
* If you are reasonably active (exercising 3-4 times each week) then you should use the higher figure in your range.
* If you are not sure, or you are somewhere in between, then your calorie intake should be somewhere in the middle of your range.

Remember to be realistic about your desired weight. You can always set new goals as you go along. You should aim for a weight that YOU feel comfortable at - a weight that will make you feel most healthful and happy.

NB: *It is not advisable to reduce your intake below 1200 calories per day - not only for health reasons (eg. daily nutritional requirements) but also to maintain your metabolic rate at an efficient fat burning level.*

Now that you know your daily calorie intake you can find out how much fat you should be consuming each day. Fats & Figures Table "B" shows you exactly how many grams of fat you can eat each day:-

Fats & Figures: Table "B"

DAILY FAT GRAM ALLOWANCE (Women & Men)			
DAILY CALORIE INTAKE	**10% FAT (grams)**	**15% FAT (grams)**	**20% FAT (grams)**
1,200	14	20	27
1,300	15	22	29
1,400	16	24	31
1,500	17	25	33
1,600	18	27	36
1,700	19	28	38
1,800	20	30	40
1,900	21	32	42
2,000	23	33	44
2,250	25	38	50
2,500	28	42	56
2,750	31	46	61
3,000	33	50	67
3,250	36	54	72
3,500	39	58	78
3,750	42	63	83
4,000	44	67	89

The above Table should be used as a guide only.

Now, using Table "B", find your daily calorie intake and look along the row to the three different figures given for fat consumption. Depending on whether you wish to maintain or lose weight, choose the relative fat percentage that I have suggested:

eg: If you are on a daily consumption of 1500 calories and you merely wish to maintain your weight, then you should follow the 20% fat gram allowance ie: 33 grams of fat each day.
However, if you wish to lose weight, then you should follow either the 10% or the 15% fat gram allowance, ie. 17-25 grams of fat each day.

TIP: If you are more than 5 kg overweight you should start on a fat reduction program of 20% for the first month or so, in order for your body and your taste buds to have time to readjust to your new way of eating. Once you begin to lose some body fat and generally when you come to within 5 kg of your goal weight (if you are extremely overweight this will obviously take more than 1 month - do not hurry it!), then you should lower your intake further - to 15%.

For those of you that have only those last stubborn 2 or 3kg to lose (I know the feeling!), then you should begin on a 15% fat intake and then reduce it to 10% after a week.

After your desired weight has been reached, you can then revert to a 20% fat intake to maintain that weight, however I have found that a constant fat intake of 10% works very well for me. (Obviously this figure may vary a little from time to time, eg. if I am on holidays and eating out a lot then I would increase it to 20%). My calorie intake is between 2,000 and 2,500 per day and I combine teaching various aerobic classes (8-9 classes each week) with swimming and weight training.

Don't forget that some fat in our diets is essential for good health and well being. You should not reduce your fat intake below the 10% level.

Also, remember to take your activity level into consideration with your daily calorie intake - the more active you are (do you exercise a lot?) the more calories you will need to consume.

If your daily calorie intake is not listed in Table B then use the following formula to calculate how many grams of fat you should eat:

1. Daily Calorie Intake x Desired Fat % = Number of calories FROM FAT that you may consume.

2. When you have the number of calories from fat that you may consume, simply divide this figure by 9 to find out how many grams of fat this equates to. (Remember 1 gram of fat equals 9 calories.)

   eg. Your Daily Calorie Intake is 1,750
   Your Desired Fat Intake % is 20%
   1,750 x 20% = 350 (calories from fat)
   350 ÷ 9 = 38.8 (grams of fat you may consume in a day)

YOUR OWN PERSONAL 'FAT BUDGET'

This is an important phrase to remember - I will refer to it occasionally throughout the book. It simply means that once you have found your daily fat intake from the Fat Allowance table (Fats and Figures Table "B"), then think of it as your 'budget' - you can spend it however you like! Yes, if you want to spend it all in one sitting, or on one meal, then you can - AND, you can choose to eat whatever foods you like within your budget.

For example: You can spend it all on breakfast, with scrambled eggs, sausages, bacon and croissants, or you may decide that you want to eat a chocolate bar at lunchtime, or visit your favourite take-away food store, or restaurant, for dinner.

If you 'blow' your budget and go over your allowance in one day then try to average out your daily allowance over two or three days.

> **eg:** If you are on an allowance of 30 grams of fat per day and on Monday you have eaten 40 grams of fat, then try to decrease your intake on Tuesday and Wednesday to 25 grams each day - making a total for the three days of 40 + 25 + 25 = 90 which will bring you back within your 'budget' of 30 grams per day (30 x 3 = 90).

You will find that although you can choose any foods that you like, you will be able to find low fat substitutes for many of your favourite foods in this book - perhaps keeping your favourites for special treats. Remember, you do not have to feel deprived.

HOW TO ADD UP YOUR 'FAT BUDGET' SCORE

All of the products listed in this book are given a serving size, either a fairly common household measure eg. 1 cup 250ml., 1 Tbsp. 20g, ¼ cup 60g, ½ can etc. or just a basic 100g serve.

Simply keep track of what you eat each day and write down the fat content by referring to the product in this book.

You will find that after a few weeks you will no longer need to write down the amounts because you will instinctively know approximately how much fat you are eating.

It is a very good idea to buy a small set of kitchen scales so that you can weigh various items if you are unsure of their exact weight.

At the end of each day, add up your score and check that you have not overspent your 'fat budget'.

NO HUNGER PANGS - EAT WHAT YOU LIKE!

By changing your everyday eating habits to a low fat regime you will never need to feel hungry again.

You will find hundreds of low fat and fat free foods that you can snack on - and if you are not overweight, then you have almost unlimited choices. However, dried fruits, jams, sugars plus some confectionery snacks, whilst containing no fat at all, are high in calorie content - so if you are trying to lose weight then you should limit these particular fat free snacks to small quantities.

Do not deprive yourself of your favourite foods - there are no forbidden foods in this low fat way of eating!

EXERCISE CONNECTION

You should combine a sensible exercise program with your new low fat way of eating. Not only will this help to promote a healthy body, it will also help to keep your metabolism moving. Your metabolism is the rate at which your body burns energy (like a motor car uses fuel). Even while you are sleeping, your body needs a certain amount of energy just to keep all of your basic bodily functions working.

Exercise can boost your metabolism, not only during exercise but also for up to 12-24 hours afterwards as well. The faster your metabolism works - the more energy (calories) it burns.

If you have not previously exercised on a regular basis then remember to start slowly. Walking is one of the best, safest and cheapest forms of exercise around. When you first start walking try to walk for 20 minutes or so at a pace that would enable you to carry on a conversation whilst doing so. In other words, you should not be out of breath.

Try to walk for 20 minutes, 3 times a week for the first few weeks and then gradually increase the length of your walk to 25 minutes, then 30 minutes, gradually building up to a 40 minute walk 3 or 4 times each week.

As your fitness level improves you will find that you will be able to increase the distance that you walk in your 40 minutes.

If walking is not to your liking then choose something else that you enjoy. The trick to sticking with an exercise program is to choose something that you enjoy doing. Variation, or 'cross training' is also another key to sticking with an exercise programme. Simply combine several different types of exercise in your programme and choose a different one each time you exercise.

eg: Monday - 40 minute walk (20 minutes beginners)
Wednesday - Aerobic dance class (Lite Pace for beginners)
Friday - 40 minute swim or bike ride or walk again.

TIP: *Don't forget to drink 6-8 glasses of water each day.*

For those of you who are perhaps already following a fairly active exercise regime (4-5 aerobic type activities each week eg. walking, cycling, jogging, swimming, dance/gym classes etc.), I suggest that you keep on with this exercise and consider adding some resistance training to your workouts.

Resistance training is simply training the body using some form of resistance. Resistance can be: your own body weight, hand held weights, circuit type machinery or the traditional weight training weights and machines.

Many people still have the stereotyped view that resistance training is only for body builders who want to 'pump iron' or athletes who wish to increase muscle size.

However, this conception is fast changing as more and more people discover the benefits of weight resistance training. Benefits which include:

* the ability to sculpt your body shape
* increased muscle tissue
* increased metabolic rate
* increased strength - ability to perform everyday tasks improves.
* stronger bones - resistance training helps slow down bone deterioration
* improved posture

When I started on a resistance training programme I saw changes in my body shape that I had not been able to achieve by doing aerobic exercise alone.

If you do incorporate a resistance training programme into your fitness regime then it is important that you have a programme designed especially for you. Most reputable fitness centres will have trained staff that will be able to assist you with a programme and also will supervise you in your workouts so that you employ the correct techniques.

Once you are started on your programme you can choose how often you would like to train (twice a week can be sufficient for general body toning) and you may decide to replace one of your aerobic exercise sessions with a resistance training one.

Resistance training will help you replace body fat with lean tissue (muscle) and thus assist in your fat loss programme. Muscle tissue burns energy (calories) and fat does not, so simply by increasing your lean body mass you will be increasing your metabolism - a double plus!

Another common misconception regarding training with weights is that women will become muscle bound 'hulks' - this is not possible unless hormonal drugs are taken. Normal weight training programmes will simply enable you to sculpt and tone your body into a more appealing shape.

Also a common myth is the idea that if you stop weight training then your muscle will 'turn to fat' - this is not possible. What will happen is that you will just lose the muscle tone and shape that you have attained.

Circuit training in fitness centres also provides a form of resistance training using special machines combined with aerobic activity. This is an excellent way to start a resistance training programme under supervision.

You would be surprised how many people of all ages, shapes and sizes are taking part in these group circuit classes now. They are very popular and you don't need a degree from a dance company to be able to participate.

Remember, it is up to you to choose which forms of exercise you enjoy doing - don't be afraid to try something new and different - you may be pleasantly surprised!

TIPS ON AVOIDING FAT FILLED FOODS

* Do not fry your foods in oil or butter - invest in a non stick pan and a can of vegetable oil spray. Dry fry, grill or oven bake (using no fat).

* Trim all fat from meat - ask the butcher to trim it before you buy it.

* Don't eat the skin on chicken - it is very high in fat.

* Replace full fat milk with a lower fat variety. Do not give up dairy products - they contain important nutritional requirements such as calcium.

  ***TIP**: If you do not like the taste of low fat or skim milk then try making your own. Buy a packet of powdered skim milk and instead of mixing it as per the directions on the packet, make it thicker and creamier by using more powder, eg. instead of mixing 1 cup of milk powder with 3 cups of water, mix 2 cups of powder instead.*

* Give up butter/margarine on your toast and sandwiches - try a fat free spread on your toast such as jam, honey or vegemite. You will be surprised at how easy it is to adapt to this taste.

* When cooking, replace sour cream with low fat natural or vanilla yoghurt - it tastes great on hot potatoes!

* Avoid deep fried take-away foods such as chips, scallops, chicken etc. *(See Recipe for Fat Free Hot Chips on Page 226)*

* When you buy tinned fish, look for the varieties packed in water or brine - not oil - not any oil!

* Limit your intake of biscuits, cakes and pastries - better still, make your own - fat free *(See Muffin recipe on page 41)*

* Keep your intake of chocolate and carob to small servings only - save for indulgences.

* When you do indulge in a high fat meal keep your portion size small - that way you can have your cake and eat it too!

* Keep your intake of eggs to 2 or 3 each week. When cooking with eggs do not use the yolk at all, just egg whites. If you prefer to not waste the egg yolks, use either a powdered egg replacer (Orgran) or frozen egg whites (Sunny Queen Just White).

* Take-Away foods: avoid pies, sausage rolls and fried foods. When ordering sandwiches ask for bread without any butter/margarine.

* Try low fat desserts such as jellies, frozen Vitari, frozen yoghurt, hot rice cream and low fat ice creams.

* Substitute a low fat cheese for full fat cheese. Devondale makes an excellent low fat cheese called 'Seven' - it is only 7% fat. (Also cooks well in sauces and even melts on toast!) Cottage cheese is also a good choice.

* Substitute low fat ice cream for full fat varieties. There are many excellent products available now that taste just as good.

* When dining out at restaurants try to order foods that are grilled or roasted instead of fried. Choose sauces that are not full of cream or butter. Avoid rich dressings and if you cannot go without dessert then order something small! Avoid the cheese platter - most of the cheeses will be high in fat.

* Don't be fooled by food labeling: LOW CHOLESTEROL DOES NOT MEAN LOW FAT, eg. Vegetable oils have no cholesterol but they are 100% fat!

* Order skim milk drinks at coffee shops eg: Cappuccino, hot chocolate.

* Avoid high fat processed meats like salami, cabanossi and pepperoni.

* Replace high fat salad dressings with a low or non fat variety - see the salad dressing section in this book for some good ideas.

* When cooking meats, soups, casseroles etc., allow them to cool until the fat solidifies and then remove it.

* Use herbs and spices to add flavour to your cooking.

* Grill, dry fry, dry bake, steam or microwave your food when cooking.

* Limit your intake of avocados. They are very high in fat (Enjoy them occasionally though, as the fat they contain is not saturated and can be quite beneficial).

* Pizza - keep serving sizes small *(see recipe for Low Fat Pizza on page 172)*.

ABBREVIATIONS

Key to Symbols and Abbreviations Used in this Book.

g	grams	strawb.	strawberry
cals.	calories	W.A.	Western Australia
ml.	millilitres	N.Z.	New Zealand
Tbsp.	tablespoon	supr.	supreme
tsp.	teaspoon	red.	reduced
w.	with	<	less than
ave.	average	wh.	whole
choc.	chocolate	oz.	ounces
ea.	each	alc.	alcohol
pcs.	pieces	decaf.	decaffeinated
cm.	centimetre	med.	medium
w'meal	wholemeal	wt.	weight
pkt.	packet	sce.	sauce
approx.	approximately	veg.	vegetables
incl.	including	eg.	for example
artif.	artificial	ctn.	carton

NB. Where measurements are given (eg: 1 cup), standard metric measures have been used.

It is a good idea to have a set of measuring cups and spoons in your kitchen, together with your kitchen scales.

1 calorie = 4.2 kilojoules

How to use 'FATs & FIGURES'

Foods are grouped in alphabetical order. Within each food section, product brands are also in alphabetical order.

Serving sizes are given for all products. You may have to adjust the figures if you use a larger or smaller serving size. This is where your kitchen scales are a necessity!

BISCUITS, CRACKERS, CRISPBREADS

These taste tempters can be a trap for those on a low fat intake - who can stop at one or two biscuits?

TIP: *When shopping for biscuits don't buy your favourite kind - instead choose a variety that you don't like as much!*

BISCUITS - CRACKERS	FAT(g)	CALS
ABUNDANT EARTH each biscuit		
Peanut Gluten Free	5.1	87
ANZAC BISCUITS each biscuit		
Home made, ave. small	3.0	60
ARNOTT'S each biscuit		
Adora Cream Wafer	1.4	28
Apricot Tartlets	2.3	58
Arno Shortbread	3.0	61
Barbeque Shapes	0.6	11
Blackberry Tartlets	2.2	57
Bran & Malt Cruskits	0.2	18
Breton/Breton salt reduced	1.0	21
Butternut Cookie	2.2	50
Cheddar Shapes	0.6	12
Cheds	2.2	39
Cheese & Bacon Shapes	0.3	8
Chicken Crimpy	0.6	13
Chilli Shapes	0.5	10
Chocolate Butternut Snap	4.1	83
Chocolate Caramel Crowns	4.3	85
Chocolate Cavetto Dark Peppermint	3.9	78
Chocolate Cavetto Milk	4.2	79
Chocolate Cherry Crowns	3.3	100
Chocolate Chip Cookie	1.8	35
Chocolate Duet	3.6	81
Chocolate Fruit & Nut	3.4	68
Chocolate Gaiety	4.0	70
Chocolate Gaiety Bar, 35g	10.6	186
Chocolate Gaiety Peanut Bar, 50g	15.6	268
Chocolate Granita	3.3	62
Chocolate Jaffa Cake	1.7	54
Chocolate Mint Slice	4.8	85
Chocolate Monte	2.7	63
Chocolate Royals Dark	2.9	73

BISCUITS, CRACKERS, CRISPBREADS

BISCUITS - CRACKERS	FAT(g)	CALS
ARNOTT'S continued ...		
Chocolate Stiks	0.5	12
Chocolate Scotch Finger	5.6	117
Chocolate Tee Vee Snacks	1.3	26
Chocolate Tim Tam	5.2	98
Chocolate Tim Tam (Caramel)	5.7	101
Chocolate Tim Tam Bar, 45g	12.7	233
Chocolate Tim Tam Hazelnut	4.6	93
Choco Saurs	2.1	50
Clix	0.9	16
Country Cheese	1.3	28
Cracked Pepper Water Cracker	0.2	12
Creamy Chocolate	3.0	72
Cruskits	0.8	28
Currant Luncheon	1.2	53
Custard Cream	3.6	75
Date Bar	1.3	65
Delta Cream	3.5	73
Farmbake Butter Shortbread	3.5	62
Farmbake Chocolate Chip	2.6	58
Farmbake Chocolate Chip Fudge	2.8	58
Farmbake Peanut Brownies	3.2	59
Full'0'Fruit	0.6	40
Gingernut (can vary from State to State)	1.0	42
Glengarry	3.8	75
Golliwog	1.6	48
Granita	2.7	60
Granita with Fruit	2.5	58
Honey Jumble	0.7	44
Honey Snaps	1.6	34
Hundreds & Thousands	0.9	42
Iced Vo Vo	1.7	59
Jatz	0.8	19
Jatz Cracked Pepper	1.0	20
Kingston	4.5	73
Lattice	2.6	52
Lemon Crisp	3.7	70
Lemon Tartlets	2.3	58
Marie	1.1	39
Maryland	3.0	56
Mediterranean Chicken Shapes	0.4	8

BISCUITS, CRACKERS, CRISPBREADS

BISCUITS - CRACKERS		FAT(g)	CALS
ARNOTT'S continued ...			
Mickey & Friends:	Chocolate	0.3	9
	Chocolate Creams	3.2	73
	Custard Creams	2.9	73
	Honey	0.4	9
Milk Arrowroot		0.9	36
Milk Coffee		1.1	40
Monte Carlo		5.0	100
Morning Coffee		0.7	26
Nice		1.9	55
Nik Nax:	Original	0.3	5
	Salt'n'Vinegar	0.2	5
Oatables		2.3	53
Orange Slice		2.8	75
Original Water Cracker		0.2	12
Pizza Shapes		0.5	9
Raspberry Shortcake		2.6	66
Raspberry Tartlets		2.4	58
Rockies 45g		12.5	228
Rye Cruskits		0.1	17
Salada		1.3	56
Salada with Multigrain		1.2	55
Salada with Wholemeal		1.2	53
Saltine		1.0	32
Sao		1.3	38
Sao with Wholemeal		1.3	37
Savoury Cheese Jatz		0.7	17
Savoury Shapes		0.4	8
Scotch Finger		4.1	86
Scotch Finger Chocolate		5.6	117
Scout Bar, 40g		8.2	169
Sesame Wheat		1.3	31
Shortbread Cream		5.2	93
Shredded Wheatmeal		1.0	33
Spicy Fruit Roll		1.0	65
Tea Cake		1.5	45
Thin Captain		0.6	23
Tina Wafer		2.4	45
Tiny Teddy/Chocolate/Honey		0.3	9
Triple Wafer		2.1	40
Venetian		3.0	66
Vita Weat, all types average		0.6	22

BISCUITS, CRACKERS, CRISPBREADS

BISCUITS - CRACKERS		FAT(g)	CALS
CADBURY'S each biscuit			
Chocolate Finger		1.3	29
Dairy Milk Wafer		4.0	69
Doubles		5.2	105
Mint Creams		2.9	79
Rainbows		4.1	86
Squiggle Tops		4.1	86
Toffee Pops		3.4	81
Zoo Animals		1.2	26
CARR'S each biscuit			
Table Water Crackers:	Regular size, each	0.6	33
	Bite Size, each	0.3	15
CLARKE'S each biscuit			
Clusters:	Apple & Walnut	6.6	144
	Apricot	3.7	112
	Banana & Peach	5.0	134
	Cherry	7.8	153
	Cherry Ripple	9.9	167
	Choc. Chip Ripple	7.4	154
	5 Fruit Muesli	6.5	145
	Fruit	7.2	149
	Fruit & Nut Ripple	8.4	159
	Oatbran Fruit & Nut	5.0	136
Cookies:	Agro	1.7	48
	Butter Rings	4.3	75
	Carob Coated Bran Treats	5.1	87
	Carob Coated Honey Snaps	4.9	86
	Charmers	4.6	85
	Choc. Delight	4.4	85
	Honey & Oat Cookies	5.2	94
	Honey Snaps	3.9	67
	Koalas	2.9	61
	Orange Shortcake	3.8	71
	Raisin & Sesame Lo Chol.	3.3	69
	Sweethearts	4.5	77
	Traffic Lights	4.0	74
Classic Cookies:	Choc Chip	4.7	90
	Dutch Speculas	3.5	78
	Golden Crunch	4.6	89

BISCUITS, CRACKERS, CRISPBREADS

BISCUITS - CRACKERS		FAT(g)	CALS
CLARKE'S continued...			
Shortbread	Classic All Butter Tails	3.8	68
	Classic Honey & Butter	3.2	58
	Classic Royal	4.8	84
FARMLAND each biscuit			
All Butter Shortbread		4.2	67
All Butter Choc. Chip Shortbread		3.7	65
Almond Crisp		4.9	86
Choc.Almond Crunch		5.1	87
Chocolate Chip/White Choc. Chip		5.2	88
Currant Crunch		5.1	87
Double Choc		5.2	88
Golden Snap		4.7	76
Hazelnut Crunch		4.7	85
Hazelnut Spice		5.2	88
Jaffa Crunch		4.5	85
Orange & Lemon Crunch		3.7	80
Peanut Crunch		4.4	85
Rainbow Nuggets		1.8	41
Rich Viennese		5.8	91
Speculas		1.9	50
Shortbread Delight		5.3	89
FREEDOM FOODS each biscuit			
Apricot & Sultana Fruit Cookie		0.7	78
Carob Rice Cookies		2.1	38
Carob Rice Crispbread, 25g each		8.0	128
Carob Rice Cakes, mini, each		2.2	75
Fruit Cookies		1.3	74
FROOKIES each biscuit			
Fruitins Fat Free, average all flavours, each		0.0	45
Fruitins Regular, all flavours, each		1.5	55
Frookies:	Animal Crackers, each	0.3	10
	Oatmeal & Raisin Cookies, each	2.0	45
	Yoghurt Cream Wafers, each	2.0	35
Frookwich Sandwich Cookies, each		2.0	50
Fat Free Crackers, all types, each		0.0	9

BISCUITS, CRACKERS, CRISPBREADS

BISCUITS - CRACKERS		FAT(g)	CALS
GLENNY'S each biscuit			
Noah & Friends Animal Cookies:	Peanut Butter	3.0	65
	Vanilla	2.0	65
	Wheat Free Oatmeal	2.0	65
GREEN'S each biscuit			
Choc Chip Cookies		2.4	60
GRIFFIN'S each biscuit			
Apricot Finger		1.1	42
Cameo Creams		3.3	79
Cameo Creams Jaffa		3.1	78
Cameo Creams Mint		3.2	78
Chit Chat		4.2	82
Chit Chat Mint		4.3	83
Choco-ade		2.6	62
Choc. Apricot Dreams		2.6	73
Chocolate Crunch		2.5	52
Chocolate Macaroon		4.3	82
Chocolate Oatmores		2.8	63
Chocolate Swiss Cream		2.3	61
Chocolate Thins		1.4	37
Chocolate Wheaten Dark		2.3	51
Chocolate Wheaten Milk		2.4	51
Dundee Shortcake		2.5	57
Fruit Finger		1.1	42
Fruit Oatmores		2.2	63
Gingernuts		1.1	55
Gingernut Bears		0.4	19
Golden Fruit		0.7	42
Hundreds & Thousands		2.2	48
Iced Vanilla Wafer		2.4	47
Jaffa Thins		1.5	38
Krispie		1.8	43
Mallowpuffs, all types		3.8	93
Malt		1.0	34
Milk Arrowroot		1.0	33
Mint Treat		4.8	86
Oatmores		2.5	64
Round Wine		0.9	28
Shell Wafer (sheet)		1.7	217

BISCUITS, CRACKERS, CRISPBREADS

BISCUITS - CRACKERS		FAT(g)	CALS
GRIFFIN'S continued...			
Super Wine		1.5	43
Striped Shortbread		3.3	66
Swiss Creme		2.6	63
Vanilla Wine		1.3	39
JACOB'S each biscuit			
Choice Grain Crackers		1.1	33
Fig Rolls		1.4	56
Lemon Puffs		4.0	81
Rich Water Biscuits		0.7	25
LANE'S each biscuit			
Apple Scrolls		2.5	60
Blueberry Mousse		3.6	79
Boston Shortbread		2.1	48
Butter Thins		1.3	29
Captain's Table:	Water	0.3	15
	Cracked Pepper	0.5	16
	Sesame	0.8	20
	Wheat	0.6	19
Chips Ahoy		2.0	50
Choc. Iced Mint		3.9	71
Choc. Mousse		2.8	72
Choco Cookie		2.3	58
Coffee Scrolls		2.3	58
Fudge Supreme		4.6	70
Gingernuts		1.1	41
Ginger Thins		1.2	29
Heyday		5.7	96
Hi Fibre Family		0.8	25
Lamington		2.5	71
Lemon Butter Thins		1.3	29
Mocha Scrolls		2.6	61
Oatmeal		1.8	45
Premium, regular		0.6	16
Premium, regular - less salt		0.5	16
Premium Lite		0.4	13
Premium Wholemeal		0.5	14

BISCUITS, CRACKERS, CRISPBREADS

BISCUITS - CRACKERS		FAT(g)	CALS
LANE'S continued			
Ritz:	Cheese/Wholemeal	1.0	17
	Plain	0.9	16
	Wheatsworth	0.6	15
Rum Slice		2.8	59
Snack Crackers:	Barbeque/Cheese	0.7	13
	Cheese & Chives/Crispy Potato	0.4	8
	Chicken	0.6	11
	Crispy Bacon	0.5	10
	French Onion	0.4	10
	Herb & Spice	0.7	14
Strawberry Cream		4.3	73
Vanilla Swirl		2.1	53
LIMMITS			
see Meal Replacers (page 173)			
McVITIE'S each biscuit			
Cheddars		1.3	21
Hob Nobs		3.1	69
Poppy & Sesame Seed Thins		1.1	20
Table Water, small		0.3	15
Wholemeal Thins		1.1	20
NATURALLY GOOD each biscuit			
Anzac Wholemeal cookies		4.5	79
Carob Rice Cake Bites, 30g		8.6	150
Coconut Crunch cookies		3.8	65
Oatbran Cookies		3.5	74
Peanut Crunch		3.8	65
NAYTURA (Safeway/Woolworths) each biscuit			
Almond & Sesame		5.0	73
Carob Coated Muesli		5.2	86
Gluten Free		3.5	66
High Fibre		4.6	65
PAMPAS Frozen Cookie Mix each biscuit			
Apricot Cookie, 30g		4.2	117
Cherry & Coconut, 30g		4.8	120
Choc. Chip, 30g		5.3	125

BISCUITS, CRACKERS, CRISPBREADS

BISCUITS - CRACKERS		FAT(g)	CALS
PARADISE each biscuit			
Cottage Cookies:	Anzac	1.7	48
	Butter Shortbread	2.9	53
	Cherry Macaroon	2.2	50
	Choc. Chip	2.0	49
	Macadamia	3.2	55
	Oat Bran & Fruit	1.7	47
	Peanut	2.4	51
	Spicy Fruit	1.7	47
Crackers:	Cheddar & Chives	0.9	22
	Cracked Pepper & Chilli	1.3	27
	Parmesan Cheese	1.2	23
	Sesame & Poppy	1.2	25
Golden Wheats:	Oat Bran	2.6	65
	Original	2.6	65
	With Fruit	2.5	65
Snacktime:	Choc. Chip Cookies	0.6	15
	Macadamia Cookies	0.9	16
	Scotch Finger	0.7	15
PHOENIX, WEBSTERS & WESTONS each biscuit			
Ace Cracker		1.2	21
Animal Munchies		1.5	33
Argyle Shortbread		1.5	33
Balmoral Cream		4.5	94
Banquet Cream		4.7	88
Bavarian Cream		3.5	65
Bikkisaurus Chocolate		0.4	9
Bikkisaurus Vanilla		0.3	9
Bites:	Cheese	0.2	6
	Cheese & Bacon	0.1	4
	Chicken	0.4	8
	Hot & Spicy	0.2	7
	Mexicana	0.2	4
	Savoury	0.4	7
Blueberry Oasis		1.8	59
Butter Shortbread Drops		1.4	31
Butternut		1.8	46
Cherry Cream		4.4	93
Choc. Animals		1.0	26
Choc & Chips		4.9	91
Chocolate Chip Cookies (Phoenix)		2.5	48

BISCUITS, CRACKERS, CRISPBREADS

BISCUITS - CRACKERS	FAT(g)	CALS
PHOENIX, WEBSTERS & WESTONS continued...		
Chocolate Chip Cookies (Westons)	1.7	37
Chocolate Cookies (Phoenix)	2.1	52
Chocolate Cookies (Westons, Websters)	1.8	46
Chocolate Cream	3.6	85
Chocolate Cream small	3.4	71
Chocolate Delight	3.1	69
Chocolate Drop Cookies	1.3	32
Chocolate Fruit Bars	4.5	115
Chocolate Jaffa	2.6	61
Chocolate Mallow Munch	4.5	120
Chocolate Mint Cream	4.3	77
Chocolate Nut Supreme	4.3	88
Choc'n'Nut Cookies	1.9	37
Chocolate Shortbread Cream	3.3	68
Chocolate Snaps	1.2	33
Chocolate Wheaten	2.9	62
Chocolate Wheaten mini	1.1	26
Cookies & Creams	3.0	63
Concerto	4.8	80
Cracker Jacks	0.8	19
Crackerbread	0.1	20
Crackerbread Wheat'n'Bran	0.2	18
Crackerbread Rye	0.1	16
Cream Assorted	3.6	81
Creamy Custard	4.4	93
Creamy Vanilla	4.4	93
Crunchy Cream	4.3	92
Custard Cream	3.3	72
Expectations	5.0	102
Family Assorted	1.7	43
Fine Fare: Choc. Chip Cookies with ginger	2.2	50
Chocolate Delight	2.2	54
Chocolate Mint Slice	6.3	110
Dark Choc. Wheats	4.0	88
Milk Choc. Wheats	4.2	89
Ginger Nut	1.1	43
Harvest Time	2.0	42
Heather Shortbread	2.7	56
Heidis	2.5	41
Highland Oatmeal	1.4	42
Honey & Malt	1.4	37

BISCUITS, CRACKERS, CRISPBREADS

BISCUITS - CRACKERS	FAT(g)	CALS
PHOENIX, WEBSTERS & WESTONS continued...		
Island Creams	5.3	84
Jam Fancies	2.4	72
Kimberley Multigrain crackers	1.0	24
Kokettes	2.6	88
La Petites	4.0	84
Lattice Shortbread	2.0	43
Lemon Cream	4.4	93
Lemon Cream small	3.2	71
Lemon Frosties	4.3	89
Lots'O'Cookies	2.2	51
Macaroon Delights	3.9	61
Malt	1.2	37
Manhattan	2.5	54
Marie	1.3	43
Mighty Mallows	2.1	80
Milk Arrowroot	1.1	36
Milk Chocolate Wheaten	2.9	62
Milk Coconut	2.4	49
Milk Coffee	1.4	41
Milk Roundabouts	2.3	62
Morning Coffee	0.9	31
Nice	1.9	55
Nursery Rhymes	1.6	37
Orange Cream	4.0	87
Peanut Cookies	2.0	48
Raspberry Oasis	1.7	58
Rich Coconut	2.2	47
Rich Shortbread	2.1	45
Rich Tea	1.3	39
Rocky Round	4.9	103
Roundabouts	2.6	63
Ryvita Original/Dark Rye	0.2	37
Ryvita Sesame Dark Rye	0.5	40
Ryvita Sesame Whole Rye	0.6	42
Scotch Fingers	2.7	56
Shredded Wheatmeal	1.6	41
Snowballs	3.5	75
St. Clemens	1.9	50
Strawberry Mallows	2.7	82
Thin Captains	0.8	25
Truffles	0.8	21

BISCUITS, CRACKERS, CRISPBREADS

BISCUITS - CRACKERS	FAT(g)	CALS
PHOENIX, WEBSTERS & WESTONS continued...		
Vanilla Cream	3.2	71
Vanilla Cream oblong	2.9	79
Vanilla Shortbread Cream	3.2	66
Village Cream Capuccino	3.3	72
Village Cream Chocolate	3.5	74
Village Cream Custard	3.6	75
Wagon Wheel	7.4	194
Wagon Wheel Mini	3.6	89
Wagon Wheel Caramel	7.5	174
Winton Water Crackers	0.5	20
PLAYER'S each biscuit		
Big Cookie, 50g each: Choc. Chunk	13.0	239
Double Choc.	13.1	238
Coconut Macaroons	1.6	32
Mini-Mates, per 30g pack: Anzac Cookies with Choc. Chips	5.5	124
Choc. Chip Cookies	7.2	132
Teddy Snacks	4.6	124
Snack Wafers: Chocolate, each	1.5	32
Vanilla, each	1.5	31
Swissh: Caramel, each	7.8	126
Chocolate/Mint, each	7.6	125
Tops: Choc./Choc. Mint, each	2.7	53
Milky/Strawberry, each	2.6	52
Wafers: Classic Vanilla, each	1.2	26
Orange Mango, each	1.2	26
Strawberry Delight, each	1.2	26
Swiss Chocolate, each	1.2	26
SUNSHINE each biscuit		
Choc. Creams	4.2	85
Choc. Crunch	1.9	47
Choc. Galore	2.8	68
Choc. Mallow Puff	3.3	75
Choc. Rice Crisps	3.8	67
Custard Creams	4.7	89
Ginger Crunch	0.8	27
Golden Cheese	0.6	20
Lemon Creams	4.4	86
Malt	1.0	33

BISCUITS, CRACKERS, CRISPBREADS

BISCUITS - CRACKERS	FAT(g)	CALS
SUNSHINE continued...		
Marie	1.1	39
Milk Coffee	1.2	39
Mr.Chips	2.0	48
Nice	1.6	43
Nutti Crunch	1.9	48
Oatmeal Crunch	2.0	48
Orange Creams	4.4	87
Toffee Crunch	1.6	47
UNIBIC each biscuit, approx		
Amaretti	1.2	35
Biscotti di Mandola	0.9	34
Cats Tongue	2.2	42
Coconut Macaroon	1.5	37
Frollini	1.8	38
Italian Shortbread	1.0	34
Viennese Crescent	2.5	44
WESTBRAE each biscuit		
Cocoa Chip Snaps	2.3	47
Cocoa Snaps	2.3	47
Carob Snaps	2.3	47
Ginger Snaps	1.7	43
Lemon Snaps	1.2	43
Oatmeal Snaps	1.7	43

BISCUITS, CRACKERS, CRISPBREADS

CRISPBREADS (each)		FAT(g)	CALS
Crackerbread, average all types		0.1	19
Cruskits:	Plain	0.8	28
	Bran & Malt	0.2	28
	Rye	0.1	17
Freedom Foods, Carob Rice Crispbread		8.3	128
Kavli		0.1	19
Olof Swedish Crisps, average		1.0	43
Orgran:	Corn Crispbread	0.1	20
	Cracked Pepper	0.2	21
Premium (Lane's) ½ whole:	Regular	0.6	16
	Lite	0.4	13
	50% less salt	0.6	16
	Wholemeal	0.4	14
Ry-Vita:	Original Whole Rye/Dark Rye	0.2	37
	No Added Salt Whole Rye	0.3	36
	Hi Fibre with Oat Bran	0.3	36
	Sesame Dark Rye	0.6	42
	Sesame Whole Rye	0.5	40
Stabburet Gourmet Thins, each:			
	with Bran & Rye	0.6	30
	with Sesame Seeds	0.7	40
	with Wheat & Oats	0.3	20
	Super Thin	1.0	70
Vita-Weat, average all types		0.6	22
Willow Valley Oat Bran		0.2	17

BREADS, BREAD ROLLS, CRUMPETS, BAGELS, MUFFINS

Bread is low in fat and provides fibre and complex carbohydrates and should make up a large part of your diet (along with fruits, vegetables and grains). Calorie and fat variations between breads are mainly due to the different weights of each type of bread.

For example: A normal sandwich slice of white bread weighs approximately 28 grams, a thick toasting slice weighs approximately 35 grams and bread rolls vary from 30 grams up to 130 grams each.

Generally: For every 30 grams of bread allow 0.7 grams of fat and 70 calories.

TIP: *Avoid high fat spreads such as butter, margarine, peanut butter etc. Opt instead for jam, honey, vegemite - all of which are fat free!*

ALL BREADS - AVERAGE	**FAT(g)**	**CALS**
Brown/Mixed Grain/Wholemeal:		
1 thin slice 30g	0.9	66
1 thick toast slice 40g	1.2	88
Damper, 1/6 20cm round loaf	6.0	300
Focaccia, 100g (15cm x 10cm slice)	7.0	300
French Bread Stick, 25g slice	0.6	56
French Toast, (dipped in egg/milk mix & fried)	6.5	165
Fruit Loaf: Light, 1 slice 30g	1.0	85
Heavy (lots of fruit), 1 slice 50g	1.8	140
Garlic Bread: ¼ French Bread Stick, 90g	17.0	370
1 slice, 20g	4.0	85
Take-Away shop, 1 roll 150g	26.0	620
Supermarket, 1 complete stick, 185g	54.0	640
1 slice, 20g	6.7	80
Lebanese Flatbread: White, 100g	2.3	271
Wholemeal, 100g	1.9	239
Lavash, 1 slice 45g	0.8	110
Pita(Pocket)Bread: Small, 60g each	0.5	150
Medium, 80-90g each	0.8	190
Pumpernickel, 1 slice 25g	0.5	47
Raisin Bread, 1 slice average 30g	1.0	80
Rice Bread, 1 slice 28g	0.7	70
Rye Bread: Dark Rye, 1 slice 30g	0.5	62
Light Rye, 1 slice 30g	0.6	73
Vienna Bread, 1 slice self cut, average 40g	1.4	105

BREADS, BREAD ROLLS, CRUMPETS, BAGELS, MUFFINS

ALL BREADS - AVERAGE		FAT(g)	CALS
White Bread:	1 sandwich slice, 28g	0.7	70
	1 toast slice, 35g	0.9	80
	1 thick self cut slice, 40g	1.0	100
	1 fibre/protein increased slice, 28g	0.8	68

TOAST: (Contains the same amount of fat & calories as the bread used.)
Remember it's the spread not the bread that has the fat!

		FAT(g)	CALS
eg.:	1 slice thin toast & 1 tsp. fat	4.7	105
	1 thick slice toast & 2 tsp. fat	8.9	150

BAGELS, BREAD ROLLS, BUNS, CROISSANTS, ROLLS

Average all brands		FAT(g)	CALS
Bagel:	medium 45g	0.7	102
	large 100g	1.4	220
	Sara Lee plain, 85g each	0.9	190
Bagel Chips & Bagel Crisps, 30g		4.0	130
Croissants, plain:	medium 50g	11.5	198
	large 70g	16.5	280
	mini 17g	4.0	68
	Sara Lee All Butter 50g each	8.5	160
Easter/Hot Cross Buns:	small 50g	2.0	140
	medium 65g	2.8	180
	large 90g	3.6	257
Fruit Bun, average 60g		2.0	150
Bread Rolls average			
Dinner roll small, 30g		0.7	70
Frankfurter/Hot dog roll, 90g		2.3	220
French roll:	small 50g	1.2	117
	large 100g	2.3	240
French bread stick, 1 slice 25g		0.6	56
Hamburger Bun:	medium 60g	1.4	140
	large 90g	2.1	210
Horseshoe roll, 60g		1.4	140
Knot roll, 60g		1.4	140
Round Sandwich Rolls:	white average 65g	1.6	153
	multigrain 65g	1.7	150
	wholemeal 65g	1.7	150
Torpedo Roll, 60g		1.4	140

BREADS, BREAD ROLLS, CRUMPETS, BAGELS, MUFFINS

BREADCRUMBS, BREAD MIXES, BREADSTICKS	FAT(g)	CALS
Basco gluten free bread mix, per 100g	0.9	325
Breadcrumbs, ½ cup, 60g	1.5	150
Breadsticks: all types, average 1 only	0.2	20
with sesame seeds, average 1 only	2.0	50
Cornflake Crumbs, ¼ cup	0.3	58
Country Harvest gluten free mix, 100g	1.0	217
Croutons: plain 15g	1.0	60
Caesar, herbed, 15g	3.0	65
Naan Bread Mix per 100g	6.7	379

CRUMPETS & MUFFINS

TIP: *Crumpets are a terrific snack - they contain next to no fat and when spread with a non fat topping such as fruit spread, vegemite, golden syrup or jam, they provide a healthy, almost fat free, low calorie treat! So stock up!*

	FAT(g)	CALS
Crumpets: average all brands, 50g each	0.5	90
Buttercup: 50g each	0.9	98
Yumpets, 30g each	0.5	60
Tip Top Golden Crumpets: 50g each	0.4	81
Golden Fingers: 36g each	0.3	59
Muffins: *(also see Cakes, page 40)*		
Buttercup: Cheese'n'Bacon, 67g each	1.7	155
English Muffin, 67g each	0.9	144
Muesli Apple Muffin, 67g each	1.3	159
Tip Top: English Muffin, 67g each	1.2	149
Multigrain Muffin, 67g each	1.7	161
Spicy Fruit Muffin, 67g each	2.0	166
Weight Watchers: 55g each	1.1	122

BREADS - VARIOUS BRANDS

BURGEN each slice	FAT(g)	CALS
Mixed Grain, 40g	1.6	96
Oat Bran & Honey, 40g	2.2	105
Rye, 40g	2.2	96
Mixed Grain Fruit, 54g	2.2	129

BREADS, BREAD ROLLS, CRUMPETS, BAGELS, MUFFINS

BREADS - VARIOUS BRANDS	FAT(g)	CALS
BUTTERCUP each slice		
Fruit'n'Spice, 34g	1.0	89
Molenberg Sandwich, 35.5g	0.9	88
Molenberg Toast, 41.5g	1.1	103
Super Sandwich Maker, 29.5g	0.7	75
Toasty (White), 34g	0.8	86
Wholemeal, 29.5g	0.7	70
Wonderwhite Sandwich, 32.4g	0.8	82
Wonderwhite Toast, 37.8g	1.0	96
COUNTRY SPLIT each slice		
Multi Grain, 24g	0.8	61
White, 24g	0.9	66
Wholemeal, 24g	0.9	60
FIELDERS each slice		
Day Bake White, 29.5g	0.7	70
Kibble 'n' Rye Toast, 34g	<1.0	78
Kibble, Rye 'n' Barley, 29.5g	0.4	70
Super Toast, 53g	1.3	125
Wholemeal, 29.5g	0.6	70
Wholemeal Toast 34g	<1.0	79
NAYTURA (Safeways/Woolworths) each slice		
White	0.7	65
White Hi-Fibre	0.7	61
Wholemeal	0.8	62
Grain	0.9	68
Light Rye	0.6	63
Oatbran & Malt	0.7	64
Unsliced Loaves: Authentic Italian, 30g slice	0.6	81
Black Rye, 50g slice	0.9	107
Full Grain Rye, 50g slice	2.8	125
Full Grain Rye & Sunflower Seed, 50g slice	2.8	125
Rye salt reduced, 50g slice	2.4	125
Schinkenbrot Rye, 50g slice	0.7	114
PRITIKIN each slice		
Whole Wheat, 30g	0.6	69
Wholemeal Toast, 30g	0.7	79
Fruit with Cinnamon, 34g	0.8	83

BREADS, BREAD ROLLS, CRUMPETS, BAGELS, MUFFINS

BREADS - VARIOUS BRANDS		FAT(g)	CALS
RIGA sliced loaves, each slice			
Black Rye, 50g		0.9	107
Danish Style Special Rye, 50g		0.5	92
Full Grain Volkornbrot, 50g		0.7	92
Funke's Rye Bread, 50g		0.7	89
Genuine Pumpernickel, 50g		0.8	96
Hamburg Style Special Rye, 50g		0.6	96
Premium Multigrain, 50g		0.8	63
Schinkenbrot, 50g		0.8	110
Schinkenbrot Special Rye, 50g		0.6	96
Sonnenkern, 50g		2.8	125
Sunflower & Barley, 42g		1.2	98
Wholemeal Light, 50g		0.5	43
TIP TOP each slice			
Bornhoffen, 30g		0.7	71
Cottage Bake:	White, 25g	0.6	61
	Multigrain, 25g	0.6	60
Dreizehn:	Rye, 39g	0.9	93
	Wholegrain Rye, 39g	0.9	79
Focaccia, 100g		3.0	242
Harvest Wholemeal with grain, 43g		1.1	100
Jumbo:	Wholemeal, 30g	0.7	69
	Toast, 35g	0.9	81
Kelly's(NSW):	Kibble'n'Rye, 28g	0.6	60
	Mighty Slice, 39g	0.8	85
	Mixed Grain, 30g	0.7	72
	Toast, 34g	0.8	74
	White, 28g	0.7	61
	Wholemeal, 30g	0.8	67
Multigrain:	Barley, 30g	0.7	71
	Malt & Honey, 30g	0.7	71
	Plain, 30g	0.7	71
	Toast, 34g	0.9	82
Spicy Fruit Loaf, 29g		0.9	75
Sunblest:	Sandwich, 30g	0.7	72
	Toast, 34g	0.9	82
Swiss Maid, 34g		0.8	82
Toast, 34g		0.8	82
White Hyfibe, 30g		0.8	70
White Hyfibe Toast, 34g		1.0	81

BREADS, BREAD ROLLS, CRUMPETS, BAGELS, MUFFINS

BREADS - VARIOUS BRANDS	FAT(g)	CALS
Tip Top each slice, continued...		
Wholemeal, 30g	0.7	69
Wholemeal Hyfibe, 30g	0.7	69
Wholemeal & Barley, 30g	0.7	69
TRÈS BON		
Average all types, Fruit/Apricot Loaf 1 slice, 1/12 whole, 58g	1.7	159
Fruit Buns, each 62.5g	1.9	171
VOGEL'S each slice		
Fruit & Nut, 41.6g	2.2	114
Honey & Oat, 41.6g	2.6	115
Light Grain, 28.3g	0.9	68
Mixed Grain & Sesame, 41.6g	2.6	109
Mixed Grain Rolls, 70g each	2.3	168
Original Swiss Grain, 41.6g	0.6	100
Sunflower & Barley, 41.6g	1.2	98
Wholemeal & Sesame, 38g	2.2	95

PITA BREADS, PIZZA BASES ETC.

		FAT(g)	CALS
Pita:	Egyptian: White, 63g	1.3	152
	Wholemeal, 63g	1.3	150
Fill-It:	White, 75g	1.4	182
	HiFibre, 75g	1.1	177
Oasis:	White, 75g	1.8	190
	Oat Fibre, 75g	1.5	190
	Lebanese White, 65g	1.3	165
	Lebanese W'Meal, 65g	1.3	163
Sahara:	White, 75g	1.3	190
	Wholemeal, 75g	1.5	188
Lavash Bread:	(pkt of 8), each 70g	2.0	204
	Yeast Free, each 70g	2.0	204
Pizza Base:	**Farmland** 430g (35cm round) incl. tomato base, 1/6 whole, 72g serve	<1.0	155
	Tip Top mini bases, 75g each	1.8	182
Mountain Bread, each square, 25g		0.4	77
Mountain Corn Bread, each square, 25g		0.3	64

BREAKFAST CEREALS

Most breakfast cereals are low in fat and are a good way to start your day. Check the packaging for salt and sugar content!

	FAT(g)	CALS
ABUNDANT EARTH		
Gluten free Muesli, 50g	3.8	181
Puffed corn, 14g	0.6	54
Puffed millet, 14g	0.4	50
Puffed rice, 14g	0.3	54
Puffed wheat, 14g	0.3	50
BRANS GENERAL average		
Barley Bran, 1 Tbsp.	0.5	31
Oat Bran, 1 Tbsp.	0.9	43
Rice Bran, 1 Tbsp.	1.6	32
Wheat Bran, unprocessed, 1 Tbsp.	0.2	11
CEROLA 30g serve		
Apricot Toasted Muesli, ¼ cup	3.1	122
Light'n'Crunchy Muesli, ¼ cup	1.7	116
Natural Muesli, ⅓ cup	2.6	114
Oat Bran Muesli, ¼ cup	2.8	118
Toasted Muesli, ¼ cup	2.8	118
DAYDAWN 40g serve		
Fruitful Apricot & Almond Porridge	1.6	160
Fruitful Fruit Medley Porridge	1.5	158
FARMLAND		
Organic Wheat Biscuits, 2 biscuits, 30g	1.0	107
Tropical Muesli, 30g	3.3	117
Tropical Toasted Muesli, 30g	4.2	124
FREEDOM FOODS 40g serve		
Muesli: Gluten Free	11.9	186
Hi Fibre	2.6	126
Natural, unsweetened	3.2	132
Yeast Free	9.2	177
GREEN'S 30g serve		
Barley Bran	1.0	92
Barley Bran Cereal	0.7	107
Barley Muesli & Fruit	1.0	107
Looney Tunes/Choc. Rings	1.9	110

GREEN'S 30g serve continued..	FAT(g)	CALS
Pebbles: Chocanilla	1.1	107
Fruity	1.2	115
Quick Barley	1.0	92
KELLOGG'S 30g serve		
All-Bran, ½ cup	0.7	110
All-Bran Fruit'n'Oats	1.0	115
Balance Flakes, 3/4 cup	1.0	119
Balance Nuggets, 1/3 cup	4.7	138
Balance Nuggets with Fruit, 1/3 cup	4.1	135
Bran Flakes, 3/4 cup	0.8	115
Coco Pops, 3/4 cup	0.1	112
Corn Flakes, 1 cup	0.4	113
Corn Pops, 1 cup	0.1	115
Crunchy Nut Corn Flakes, 3/4 cup	1.2	118
Frosties, 3/4 cup	0.3	116
Fruit Loops, 1 cup	1.3	121
Honey Smacks, 3/4 cup	0.2	116
Just Right, 1/3 cup	0.4	114
Komplete Muesli Natural, ¼ cup	0.9	111
Komplete Muesli Oven Baked, ¼ cup	3.1	125
Mini-Wheats: Whole Wheat: 1 cup	0.8	113
Apricot/Blackcurrant, ½ cup	0.4	112
Nutri-Grain, 1 cup	0.8	118
Oat'n'Honey Bake, 1/3 cup	2.1	137
Puffed Wheat, 1¼ cups	0.7	120
Rice Bubbles, 1 cup	0.1	112
Special K, 1 cup	0.2	114
Sultana Bran, 2/3 cup	0.3	111
Sustain, ½ cup	0.9	120
LOWAN FOODS 30g serve		
Barley Flakes	0.5	106
Muesli: Natural	1.7	109
Tropical Gold Natural	2.5	103
Natural Wheat Germ	2.3	114
Oat Bran	1.5	114
One Minute Oats	2.6	118
Rice Flakes	0.6	108
Rolled Oats/Traditional	2.6	118
Rye Flakes	0.5	106

BREAKFAST CEREALS

	FAT(g)	CALS
MORNING SUN		
Muesli: Apricot & Almond, 60g	4.4	209
Peach & Pecan, 60g	4.1	209
Tropical Toasted, 60g	8.8	253
NAYTURA 30g serve		
Barley Bran Flakes	0.5	105
Barley Flakes	0.5	105
NORGANIC CRUNCHOLA 30g serve		
Average all varieties	<1.0	94
OATS - ROLLED OATS GENERAL average		
Dry, 1 Tbsp., 10g	0.9	35
¼ cup, 30g	2.7	115
Porridge (with water) 1 cup, 245g	2.5	122
Porridge (with 50% water/50% milk) 1 cup, 245g	5.5	150
OLD GRAIN MILL 30g serve		
Bran, natural	1.4	48
Muesli: Australian Gold Tropical Fruit	1.9	111
Australian Gold Toasted Tropical Fruit	2.3	118
Classic	2.6	115
Fruit & Nut	2.5	112
Natural	1.7	109
Oat Bran	2.6	115
Quick Cooking Oats	3.3	117
Rolled Oats/Traditional	2.6	117
OLYMPIC 30g serve		
Muesli: Apricot & Almond, ¼ cup	2.3	107
Tropical, ¼ cup	1.5	110
Walnut & Mango, ¼ cup	3.4	119
ONLY NATURAL 30g serve		
Breakfast Crunch	2.1	120
Ricebran	6.0	132
PROVITA		
Wheat Hearts, 30g	2.0	93
PURINA		
Fruit'n'Bran Flakes, 45g	1.1	140
Muesli Cornflakes, 45g	0.8	169
Processed Bran, 45g	1.5	141
Shredded Wheat, 25g	0.3	86

BREAKFAST CEREALS

PURINA continued..	FAT(g)	CALS
Swiss Muesli, 60g	4.7	216
Toasted Muesli, 60g	10.7	267
Toasted Muesli Flakes, 45g	2.3	163
Unprocessed Bran, 12g	0.7	27
SANITARIUM 30g serve		
Bran Bix, 2 = 30g	1.2	89
Bran Cereal	2.5	80
Corn Flakes, approx. 1¼ cups	0.4	110
Crunchy Bix, 2 = 30g	1.6	111
Fruity Bix, Apricot/Tropical	0.6	105
Good Start, 2 = 30g	1.8	108
Granola: Natural, ²/₃ cup	0.7	105
Crunchy, ¼ cup	6.3	132
Granose	0.8	101
Honey Weets, 1½ cups	0.8	110
Light'n'Tasty	1.2	105
Lite Bix, 2 = 30g	0.8	101
Muesli: Natural, ¼ cup	1.4	105
Unsweetened, ¼ cup	2.6	110
Golden Toasted, ¼ cup	7.0	140
Oats 1 minute	2.7	113
Puffed Wheat, 1½ cups	0.8	108
Ricies, 1½ cups	0.4	111
San-Bran, ¹/₃ cup	2.5	80
Traditional Oats	2.7	113
Weet Bix, 2 = 30g	0.8	100
Weet Bix Hi Bran, 2 = 40g	2.9	132
Weet Bix Oat Bran, 2 = 40g	1.9	138
Wheat Germ, 1 Tbsp., 8g	2.4	102
SUNFARM 30g serve		
4 Brans	3.2	124
Ricebran	6.0	132
UNCLE TOBY'S 30g serve		
Choc Dot Crispies	0.7	118
Clusters Oven Baked Muesli	4.9	129
Crunchy Oat Bran	1.7	113
Crunchy Oat Bran with Fruit	1.3	107
Crunchy Oat Flakes	2.6	106
Fibre Plus	0.9	99
Hi Fibre Oats	2.4	110

BREAKFAST CEREALS

UNCLE TOBY'S 30g serve, continued..		FAT(g)	CALS
Instant Porridge Plus		1.7	115
Kornie Cornflakes		0.2	108
Lite Start		0.3	103
Muesli:	Natural Swiss	2.2	106
	Natural Apricot & Almond	2.2	105
	Flakes	0.7	105
Oat Bran		2.6	110
Oatflakes		1.3	115
Rice Crispies		0.8	115
Shredded Wheat, 1 biscuit, 25g		0.3	80
Sportplus		0.8	106
Sultanas'n'Wheat Bran		1.1	100
Traditional Oats		2.3	111
Vita Brits Organic, 2 biscuits, 30g		0.5	104
Weeties plain		0.4	104
Weeties Fruit'n'Nut		0.9	105
Wheat Bites		0.9	105
Breakfast Bars, each:	Lite Start	2.3	135
	Fibreplus	3.0	172
	Sports Plus	2.5	145
Clusters each, 60g		9.5	248
WEIGHT WATCHERS			
Fruit & Fibre, 20g, 1/3 cup		0.8	107
Tropicana, 30g, 1/3 cup		0.5	108
WHEATGERM			
All brands, 1 Tbsp., 6g		0.4	16
WILLOW VALLEY 30g serve			
Agro's cocoa bubbles, 1 cup		1.3	122
Barley O's, 1 cup		0.7	111
Cocoa Bombs, 1 cup		1.3	122
Corn Bubbles, 1 cup		0.6	108
Fing O's, 30g		2.5	127
Hi-Fibre Corn Flakes, 1 cup		0.5	115
Honey O's, 1 cup		1.6	121
Multi Bran, 2/3 cup		2.7	123
Oat Bran, ½ cup		2.9	113
Rice & Oat Bran Bubbles, 1 cup		0.2	111
Oat Bran Crunchy, Toasted, ½ cup		2.9	113
Slam Dunks, 30g, 1 cup		1.0	111

CAKES & DESSERTS

Most cakes and desserts contain a high percentage of fat.
Save them for the occasional indulgence!

Note: Figures given are estimates only and will obviously vary from each retail/coffee shop/take away outlet etc.

TIP: *Angel Cake and Meringue (plain) have no fat.*

CAKES - FRESH	**FAT(g)**	**CALS**
Angel Cake, 1/10 20cm. round cake	0.0	181
Apple Cake, 1/8 20cm. round cake	7.5	190
Apple Pie: individual, average, 125g	17.0	330
McDonald's, 87g	17.5	274
1/8 home made, approx. 100g	15.0	250
Apple Strudel (puff pastry) average serve	20.0	400
Banana Cake, 1/8 20cm. round cake	15.0	330
Black Forest Cake, 100g	19.0	350
Brandy Snaps, 1 cream filled	11.5	170
Butter Cake 1/8 20cm. round cake	15.0	330
Carrot Cake, iced:		
Coffee Shop 5cm x 5cm x 5cm (100g)	20.0	315
Homemade 1/12 20cm. round cake, (130g)	26.0	400
Cheesecake: small slice, 60g	13.0	208
large slice, 130g	29.0	450
Chocolate Brownie, 40g	12.0	183
Chocolate Cake - Homemade/Block:		
plain 1/10 20 cm. round cake, 60g:	11.0	227
plus frosting (no fat), ADD	0.0	50
plus chocolate/butter icing, ADD	4.0	50
plus cream filled, ADD	4.0	75
Chocolate Eclair with filling	18.0	271
Chocolate Fudge, 70g slice	21.0	320
Chocolate Gateau (coffee shop) 1/8 cake, large slice, 100g	26.0	450
Chocolate Mud Cake: small slice, 50g	13.0	225
large slice, 100g (1/8 whole cake)	26.0	450
Christmas Cake, average, 60g slice	6.5	194
Coconut Macaroon, 1 only	6.0	130
Coconut Slice 50g - 5cm x 5cm x 2cm.	6.0	156
Cream Bun, 1	18.0	225
Cream Horn, 65g	23.5	280
Cream Puff with custard filling, 100g	15.0	243
Croissant: average, 70g each	16.0	274
mini, 17g each	4.0	67

CAKES & DESSERTS

CAKES - FRESH

	FAT(g)	CALS
Cupcake, plain, 1 only	3.0	90
Iced, 1 only	6.0	140
Custard Tart, 135g	18.0	360
Danish Pastry, average 100g	15.5	311
Date & Walnut Loaf, 75g slice	7.0	225
Doughnut: Plain (Cinnamon/Sugar) each	10.3	187
Iced, each	13.0	260
Cream & Jam filled, each	19.5	350
Eclair, Chocolate with filling, each	18.0	271
Finger Bun, iced (unbuttered), 1, 65g	5.0	192
Florentine, 1	7.5	160
Fruit Bun: glazed, 60g	2.0	150
iced, 75g	6.0	225
Fruit Cake: Rich, 50g slice	6.0	210
Light (less fruit), 50g slice	7.3	170
Fruit Mince Pie	10.0	230
Fruit Mince Slice, iced 150g	14.0	445
Fruit Pies: Homemade 1/6 pie, 135g	19.0	320
(All fruit incl. Apricot, Boysenberry, Blueberry, Blackberry, Loganberry, Gooseberry).		
Galactobureko (Greek Pastry)	14.0	342
Gingerbread, average 80g	5.8	230
Hazelnut Torte, 1/10 whole	30.0	400
Hot Cross Bun/Easter Bun	2.8	180
Jam Tart, 1, 50g	7.4	175
Lamington: small 50g	6.0	160
medium 75g	9.0	240
cream & jam centre, 75g	13.0	270
Lemon Chiffon Pie, 115g slice	14.0	340
Lemon Meringue Pie, 1/8 23cm. round pie	12.0	310
Macaroon, Almond, 1	6.0	130
Madeira Cake, 60g slice	9.0	220
Marble Cake, 60g slice	9.0	220
Meringue, 1, 25g	0.2	95
'Mushroom' tartlet, 1,	7.5	200
Pecan Pie, 1/10 23cm. round pie	26.0	414
Plain Cake, Homemade/Block:		
(incl. Vanilla, Lemon, Orange, Cinnamon, Coffee)		
Plain 1/10 20cm, round cake, 60g:	11.0	225
plus Frosting (no fat) ADD	0.0	50
plus Chocolate/Butter Icing ADD	4.0	50
plus Cream Filled ADD	4.0	75

CAKES & DESSERTS

CAKES - FRESH		FAT(g)	CALS
Profiterole, Chocolate/Caramel, 1		14.0	198
Rock Cake, large, plain, 1		8.0	250
Scones:	Plain/Fruit (no fat), 1, 40g	4.0	125
	plus butter	8.0	160
	plus butter & jam	8.0	185
	plus cream & jam	12.0	225
Scone Mix (White Wings) average serve, 30g		2.0	75
Sponge:	1/8 20cm round cake, 50g	2.5	145
	1/8 20cm round cake jam & cream filled	8.0	195
	Whole Cake eg. **Top Taste**, 350g	19.6	1170
Sultana Cake, 50g		7.5	175
Swiss Roll ave. all types, 40g		2.5	125
Tea Cake, plain 40g		3.0	120
Vanilla Slice, average 135g		12.0	275

MUFFINS - CAKE TYPE averages only (Coffee Shop/Cake Shop etc.)		FAT(g)	CALS
Apple & Cinnamon, Apricot, Blueberry:			
	1 Medium 60g	7.4	160
	1 Large 100g	12.3	260
	1 Extra Large 150g	18.5	390
Banana & Raisin:			
	1 Medium 60g	7.4	173
	1 Large 100g	12.3	289
	1 Extra Large 150g	18.5	428
Bran & Date:			
	1 Medium 60g	7.4	145
	1 Large 100g	12.3	240
	1 Extra Large 150g	18.5	385
Chocolate Chip:			
	1 Medium 60g	8.5	170
	1 Large 100g	14.0	282
	1 Extra Large 150g	21.0	420
Date & Walnut:			
	1 Medium 60g	8.3	172
	1 Large 100g	13.7	287
	1 Extra Large 150g	20.6	425
Homemade - Using no fat or sugar: *(see recipe next page)*			
	1 Medium 60g	0.3	90
	1 Large 100g	0.5	130
McDonald's Apple/Oatbran Muffin, 75g		2.1	195

CAKES & DESSERTS

Karen's Fat Free Muffins

You will love these muffins and you can experiment with your own variations. You can exchange any of the fruit for other fruits and you can also use low fat plain or flavoured yoghurt instead of the apple sauce. If you wish you can add some nuts, however you will then need to add the fat and calorie contents of the nuts to your muffins.

Basic Mix

2 cups S.R. wholemeal flour
¼ cup bran
¼ cup Splenda (you can use sugar if you prefer - just add the extra calories).
1 cup raisins or sultanas
1½ cups frozen or fresh blueberries
1 very ripe banana
¾ cup apple sauce
1½ cups skim milk
2 egg whites or 2 tsp. egg replacer
1 Tbsp. baking powder

Method

In one bowl mix the flour, baking powder, raisins, Splenda and blueberries.

In a blender (or another bowl) mix the banana, skim milk, apple sauce and the egg whites. Then add this mixture to the flour mixture and mix well.

Pour into a muffin tray (pre sprayed with a vegetable oil spray) and bake in a moderate oven for 15-18 mins. (do not overcook or they will dry out).

Yield

I usually make 18 muffins from this mix:	Each Muffin	0.3g fat	90 cals
If you only make 12 muffins:	Each Muffin	0.5g fat	130 cals

CAKES & DESSERTS

DESSERTS - FRESH	FAT(g)	CALS
Apple Charlotte, average serve	12.0	450
Apple Crumble, (½ cup), 150g	9.0	200
Apple Flan, 1/6 20cm. flan	16.0	450
Apple Pie *(see Cakes page 38)*		
Apple Strudel *(see Cakes page 38)*		
Banana Split (with cream & ice cream)	32.0	600
Blancmange, average serve, 125g	4.8	150
Bombe Alaska, 1/8 whole	16.0	340
Bread & Butter Pudding, average serve	18.0	365
Bread Pudding, average serve, 110g	9.5	325
Charlotte Russe, average serve	20.0	420
Chocolate Mousse, small, 80g	18.0	200
Chocolate Pudding, steamed, average serve	15.0	350
Chocolate Sauce, ¼ cup	5.8	155
Chocolate self-saucing pudding (see Puddings)		
Coconut Custard, 150g	20.0	293
Custard: Baked, ½ cup	6.5	129
Baked, ½ cup with skim milk/artif. sweetener.	0.0	64
Egg Custard, ½ cup 125g	6.0	140
Custard pie, 150g	23.0	400
Custard Powder: dry 1 Tbsp., 10g	0.0	35
Prepared ½ cup	4.0	117
Prepared with low fat milk, ½ cup	2.5	101
Prepared with non fat milk, ½ cup	0.0	90
Lemon Chiffon Pie, 115g serve	14.0	340
Lemon Meringue Pie, 1/8 23cm. pie	12.0	310
French Fruit Flan, glazed 1/10 23cm flan	8.0	200
Fruche *(see Dairy Desserts page 44)*		
Frozen Yoghurt *(see Ice Confections page 121)*		
Fudge Sundae, 165g	8.0	265
Golden Syrup Dumplings, each	6.5	172
McDonald's: Apple Pie, 87g	17.5	274
Cookies, 60g each	12.5	290
Apple/Oatbran muffin, 75g	2.1	195
Hot Fudge Sundae, 163g	8.2	265
Hot Caramel Sundae, 163g	8.2	265
Pavlova: with fruit & cream, 1/12 30cm pavlova	8.0	220
Shells Only: average, 40g weight	0.0	130
Giant Shell 500g	0.0	1600
Individual Shell 100g	0.0	325
Ezi-Pav **(Green's)** dessert mix, 100g	0.0	269

CAKES & DESSERTS

DESSERTS - FRESH	FAT(g)	CALS
Peach Melba, average serve, 1 peach	6.8	350
Pecan Pie, 1/10 23cm. pie	22.0	385
Plum Pudding, Christmas (rich), ½ cup	10.0	400
Puddings: Chocolate, steamed, average serve	15.0	350
Self Saucing sponge, average:		
Chocolate, 100g	2.9	160
Lemon, 100g	3.3	180
Other flavours, 100g	1.3	145
Big Sister self saucing sponge puddings:		
(Tinned per 108g serve): Golden	8.7	310
Butterscotch	8.3	307
Chocolate	12.9	337
Rice Puddings/Creamed Rice:		
Canned average all brands, Vanilla, 150g	3.5	180
Parsons: Vanilla, 150g	2.1	122
Apricot, 150g	8.9	160
Banana, 150g	9.5	165
Chocolate, 150g	4.4	140
Ambrosia Low Fat, 150g	0.8	113
Sorbet, average serve, 150g	0.0	100
Strawberry Shortcake/Cream, 1/6 20cm cake	15.0	360
Tapioca Cream, home made average serve	10.0	260
Trifle, 120g	11.0	206
Upside Down Cake, 1/8 whole	9.5	180

CREPES, PANCAKES, PIKELETS, WAFFLES		
Crepes, plain, each, 20cm.	1.5	70
Crepes Suzette, 2	20.0	400
Griddle Cakes (corn), 75g each	6.5	157
Griddle Cakes (flour), 50g each	8.0	136
Pancakes, plain average all types: Large, 75g, 20cm.	5.0	100
Medium, 50g, 15cm.	3.5	70
Pancake Mix (**White Wings, Panjacks**)		
50g, made as directed	2.3	95
Pancake Shake (**Green's**), 50g, made as directed:	1.0	85
Apple & Cinnamon, Original	1.6	187
Banana, Blueberry	1.7	188
Choc. Chip	4.9	204
Pikelets, pre packaged 1, 12g	1.0	37
homemade, 1, 20g	1.7	60
Waffles, average 1	5.0	120

CAKES & DESSERTS

DAIRY DESSERTS	FAT(g)	CALS
Ambrosia Devon Custard, 100g	3.1	102
Cadbury Mousse, 85g ctn: Dairy Milk	6.8	160
Peppermint Chocolate	7.1	162
White Chocolate	7.5	154
Creamed Rice: average, 150g, vanilla	3.5	180
Jacaranda, 150g	2.7	153
Parsons: Vanilla, 150g	2.1	122
Apricot, 150g	8.9	160
Banana, 150g	9.5	165
Chocolate, 150g	4.4	140
Ambrosia, Low Fat ,150g	0.8	113
Dairy Custards:		
Australian Farmers Brandy Custard, 100ml.	2.0	84
Caboolture/Australian Farmers, 100ml.	2.0	84
Caboolture Snack Pack, 200g pkt.	4.4	188
Dairy Farmers, 100ml.	2.9	98
Dairy Farmers UHT Vanilla, 100ml.	3.2	102
Dairy Lite low fat, 100ml.	0.9	80
Dubbel Vla, 100ml.	2.2	98
Garden City, 100ml.	3.3	92
Jacaranda Vanilla, 100ml.	2.2	94
Nimbin Low Fat, 100ml.	0.2	81
Oak UHT Vanilla, 100ml.	2.8	98
Oak UHT Chocolate, 100ml.	2.8	98
Unity Vanilla, 100ml.	2.0	84
Danone Sprinklins' 117g ctn.: Chocolate	4.8	183
Strawberry	3.7	171
Dany, 150g ctn: Chocolate	6.6	211
Choc-Caramel	6.3	205
Banana, Strawberry, Vanilla	5.1	190
Encore (Browne's W.A.), 200ml ctn.:		
Berry Fruits	4.5	236
Chocoballs	8.7	273
Muesli	6.2	280
Strawberry, 170ml.	4.5	234
Fromais (Kraft), 175g ctn: Apricot Delight	7.0	210
French Vanilla	7.6	216
Forest Berries	7.0	216
Mango/Passionfruit	7.0	221
Wild Strawberry	7.0	221
Fruche: average all flavours, 200g ctn	8.0	230
Low Fat/Light per 200g ctn.	1.0	125

CAKES & DESSERTS

DAIRY DESSERTS		FAT(g)	CALS
Garden City:	Caramel Dairy Dessert, 200g ctn	5.2	105
	Chocolate Dairy Dessert, 200g ctn	5.2	108
	Vanilla-Choc. 200g ctn.	5.2	105
Gise Creme Glace soft serve, 100g		0.0	30
Norco, low chol. frozen, 50g		4.8	102
Peter's Farm:	Creme Caramel, 150g ctn.	6.9	197
	Creme Chocolate, 150g ctn.	7.0	198
	Chocolate Mousse, 150g ctn.	11.9	285
Yogo, 200g ctn.:	Banana	5.3	250
	Chocolate	6.1	263
	Strawberry	5.2	249
Snak Pak (Foster Clark's), 150g tub, average:			
	Banana, Chocolate, Strawberry, Vanilla	5.0	195
	Caramel, Double Chocolate average	5.4	195

VARIOUS BRANDS - PACKET, FRESH & FROZEN

		FAT(g)	CALS
ABUNDANT EARTH			
Brown Rice Baking Mix, 100g		4.5	335
Buckwheat Pancake Mix, 100g		2.5	340
BASCO			
Gluten Free Bread Mix, 100g		0.9	325
Gluten Free Vanilla Cake Mix, 100g		9.4	396
BETTY CROCKER made up as directed			
Bisquik: Variety baking mix, 1 cup		8.0	240
Brownie Mix 1 brownie:	Fudge Brownie	9.0	200
	Frosted Brownie	6.0	160
	Hot Fudge Supreme Brownie	7.0	140
Cake Mixes, made as directed, 1/12 whole cake:			
Supermoist:	Angel Cake (Fat Free)	0.0	140
	Choc. Fudge Cake	12.0	260
	Devil's Food Cake	12.2	250
	French Vanilla	11.1	250
	Madeira	9.0	200
	Marble	11.0	260
	Marble No Cholesterol	7.0	220
	Milk Chocolate	12.0	260
	Milk Chocolate No Cholesterol	7.0	210

CAKES & DESSERTS

VARIOUS BRANDS - PACKET, FRESH & FROZEN	FAT(g)	CALS
BETTY CROCKER continued...		
Frosting Mixes, 2 Tbsp., 34g: Dark Dutch Fudge	6.0	160
Milk Chocolate	6.0	160
Vanilla	5.0	140
Muffin Mixes, made as directed, each muffin:		
Apple Cinnamon	4.0	140
Apple Cinnamon No Cholesterol	3.0	130
Banana Nut	5.0	150
Banana Nut No Cholesterol	4.0	140
Blueberry	5.0	170
Blueberry No Cholesterol	3.0	150
BIG SISTER		
Low Fat Cakes, 50g, 1/5 cake:		
Chocolate	1.5	138
Orange	1.4	145
Vanilla	1.5	150
Nature Cakes, 44g serve, 1/8 cake:		
Banana & Pecan	11.0	187
Carrot	10.6	188
Date & Pecan	9.5	184
Honey & Oat	10.8	191
Pumpkin	10.6	193
Self Saucing Puddings (tinned), 108g serve:		
Butterscotch	8.3	307
Chocolate	12.9	337
Golden	8.7	310
BIRDS		
Angel Delight, made as directed, 1/4 pkt.:		
Banana/Caramel	6.0	110
Chocolate/Mint Chocolate	5.6	105
Chocolate with Choc. Chips	6.8	142
Strawberry	6.2	110
BON GATEAUX Frozen Desserts		
Bavarians: Capuccino, 1/6 whole, 75g	16.5	253
Chocolate, 1/6 whole, 75g	15.3	234
Cheesecakes: 1/6 whole, 75g:		
French	13.5	225
Pineapple, Passionfruit & Cream	15.5	227
Strawberries & Cream	13.8	206

CAKES & DESSERTS

VARIOUS BRANDS - PACKET, FRESH & FROZEN	FAT(g)	CALS
COUNTRY HARVEST		
Gluten free, multi-purpose baking mix, 100g	3.9	367
DANISH LUXURY CAKES		
1/6 whole, 50g: Almond Marzipan	4.5	79
Kiwi	4.2	74
Marble Marmor	5.1	84
Strawberry	4.2	74
DEFIANCE		
Nature's Kitchen, made as directed:		
Chocolate Cake Mix, 1/12 whole	3.6	105
Chocolate Slice Mix, 1/12 whole	13.3	206
Cookie Mixes, average each cookie, 12g:		
Anzac Biscuits	3.5	58
Choc. Chip Cookies	2.7	56
Apricot & Muesli Slice, 50g	8.3	219
Scone Mix, made as directed, average each scone	1.2	45
Shake & Pour Pancake Mixes, 50g serve average all flavours	0.7	97
Shake & Pour Dessert Mixes, 100g serve, Chocolate	6.5	183
Yoghurt Icing Mix, 1 Tbsp., 25g	1.2	83
DEFIANCE - PYMBLE KITCHEN FROZEN DESSERTS		
1/8 whole: Apple Crumble, 62.5g	7.6	200
Apricot Crumble, 62.5g	8.0	195
Blueberry Crumble, 62.5g	7.4	183
Macadamia Nut Pie, 56.2g	15.7	250
Pecan Pie, 56.2g	15.4	247
FARMLAND		
Fresh Packaged Cakes, Slices, Muffins:		
Apricot Napolean Slice, 29g each	4.3	114
Coconut Slice, 38g each	7.4	147
Fairy Cakes: Jam, each	4.1	104
Sultana, each	3.6	104
Wholemeal, each	3.9	99
French Tea Cake, 1/10 whole, 35g	5.6	127
Fruit Cake: Light 1/16 whole, 50g	5.8	170
Dark, 1/16 whole, 50g	6.1	173
Fruit Mince Pies, each	7.5	193
Golden Sponge, 1/12 whole, 34g	1.7	101

VARIOUS BRANDS - PACKET, FRESH & FROZEN	FAT(g)	CALS
FARMLAND continued...		
Iced Banana Sponge Fingers, each	4.1	100
Iced Passionfruit Sponge Fingers, each	4.1	100
Jam Butter Cookies, 12.5g each	3.6	63
Lemon Butter Cookies, 12.5g each	3.6	64
Lamington Jam Fingers, 30g each	3.1	101
Lamington Jam & Cream Fingers, 29g each	5.2	112
Lamingtons, 58g each	6.0	195
Madeira: Plain, 1/10, whole, 35g	5.1	122
Chocolate, Iced, 1/10 whole, 40g	5.2	142
Orange, Iced, 1/10 whole, 40g	5.4	143
Muffins: Apple & Spice, 75g each	18.5	296
Apple & Spice mini, 22g each	5.4	87
Blueberry, 75g each	18.8	310
Blueberry mini, 22g each	5.5	91
Sultana & Oatbran, 75g each	18.2	331
Sultana & Oatbran mini, 22g each	5.3	97
Napolean Slice, 29g each	4.3	114
Rainbow Layer Sponge, 1/10 whole, 38g	5.7	139
Rollettes: Chocolate, 42g each	9.7	172
French, 42g each	5.7	149
Jam, 42g each	1.9	129
Sponge Roll: Jam, 1/10 whole, 32g	1.6	94
Chocolate/Cream Filled, 1/10 whole, 32g	6.9	123
Squiggles, 50g each	8.1	192
Sultana Cake: Plain, 1/10 whole, 35g	3.6	112
Iced, 1/10 whole, 40g	4.8	135
Frozen Cakes, Gateaux & Desserts:		
Apple Pie, 1/6 whole, 100g	10.7	238
Bavarian, 1/6 whole, 75g: Capuccino Cream	15.7	243
Choc. Cream	16.5	252
Choc. Mint	15.4	236
Cheese Cake, 1/6 whole:		
Original, 83g	14.9	241
Pineapple, Passionfruit & Cream, 75g	12.8	205
Strawberries & Cream, 75g	13.3	219
Danish, 1/6 whole: Apple, 67g	6.9	159
Blueberry, 67g	5.9	176
Pecan Pie, 1/6 whole, 75g	20.3	322
Traditional Apple Strudel, 1/5 whole, 100g	13.1	250

CAKES & DESSERTS

VARIOUS BRANDS - PACKET, FRESH & FROZEN	FAT(g)	CALS
FRENCH KITCHEN		
Choc-Coated Profiteroles, each	5.1	93
GREEN'S		
Cake Mixes, 1/12 whole, 50g, made as directed:		
Banana	4.7	161
Carrot	11.2	233
Chocolate	4.2	136
Date Loaf	2.8	130
Dark Chocolate	5.9	185
Golden Butter	9.4	207
Madeira Sultana	6.5	150
Swiss Milk	9.6	185
Shake-a-Cake, 50g serve		
Carrot	8.5	160
Chocolate	7.6	150
Orange	8.0	161
Madeira	7.7	155
Sultana Butter	7.5	153
Choc. Chip Cookies, 12g each	2.4	60
Microbake 100g: Apricot	12.5	251
Chocolate	12.1	234
Dessert Mixes, made up as directed:		
Chocolate Mousse, 100g	6.1	130
Ezi-Pav Pavlova, 100g	0.0	269
Original Cheesecake, 100g	19.2	315
Muffin Mix, each muffin, 60g, made as directed:		
Banana	9.4	186
Blueberry	9.6	189
Honey & Walnut	9.8	185
Pumpkin & Spice	8.8	171
Pancake Shake, 50g, made as directed:	1.0	85
Apple & Cinnamon, Original	1.6	187
Banana, Blueberry	1.7	188
Choc. Chip	4.9	204
Self Saucing Sponge Puddings, 100g, made as directed:		
Chocolate	2.9	160
Lemon	3.3	181
Apple & Cinnamon, Apricot	1.3	145
Butterscotch & Forestberry	1.3	145

CAKES & DESSERTS

VARIOUS BRANDS - PACKET, FRESH & FROZEN	FAT(g)	CALS
MOTHER EARTH		
Fresh cakes:		
Apricot & Raisin, 1/10 whole, 45g	2.3	134
Magdalenas, each: Apricot	6.3	152
Chocolate	8.7	172
Strawberry	7.8	159
Wholemeal Fruit Bar, 50g	2.4	170
Wholemeal Raisin Bar, 50g	2.4	170
MR. KIPLING		
Fresh cakes, each cake/slice:		
Almond slice, 32g	4.7	143
Battenberg Treats, 35g	6.8	176
Bramley Apple & Custard Pies	10.1	254
Cherry Bakewell, 46g	8.6	218
French Fancies, 25g	2.9	107
Jaffa Fingers, 24g	6.9	136
Glazed Mince Tartlets, each	8.3	226
Mince Pies, each	9.1	253
Rich Chocolate Slice, 31g	6.1	144
NANNA'S		
Family Fruit Pies:		
Apple, 1/6 pie, 100g	10.3	230
Apple Light, 1/6 pie, 100g	7.0	202
Apple Big Bake, 1/8 pie, 100g	9.3	203
Apricot, 1/6 pie, 100g	10.1	233
Blackberry & Apple, 1/5 pie, 100g	10.4	260
Cinnamon Apple, 1/6 pie, 100g	10.3	235
Rhubarb & Apple, 1/6 pie, 100g	10.3	257
Tropical Dessert, 1/5 pie, 100g	11.3	310
Snack Pies, each:		
Apple, 125g	15.4	334
Apricot, 112.5g	13.4	297
Blackberry & Apple, 112.5g	13.4	305
Blueberry & Apple, 112.5g	13.4	305
Strudels: ¼ whole, 100g:		
Apple	11.7	253
Blueberry & Apple	13.3	260
Sultana Creme	18.7	350

CAKES & DESSERTS

VARIOUS BRANDS - PACKET, FRESH & FROZEN	FAT(g)	CALS
NANNA'S continued...		
Apple Rolls, 29.2g each	3.3	69
Waffles, each: Blueberry	1.0	48
Double Choc.	1.6	53
Original	1.2	46
PAMPAS:		
Apple Strudel, ¼ whole, 105g	3.8	395
Cookie Mix, each cookie, 30g: Apricot	4.2	117
Cherry & Coconut	4.8	120
Choc. Chip	5.3	125
Fruit Twirls: Apricot, ¼ pkt, 112.5g	12.2	275
Boysenberry, ¼ pkt, 112.5g	12.2	275
Strawberry, ¼ pkt, 112.5g	12.2	275
Lattice Puffs: Apricot, 50g	4.2	128
Apple, 50g	5.4	138
Lemon Meringue Pie, 1/6 pie, 75g	6.5	186
Puffs, average all flavours, each puff	5.6	130
PUFFIN		
Self Saucing Sponge Puddings, 1/6 pkt, 100g, made as directed: average all flavours	3.0	190
SARA LEE		
Bagels, plain, 85g each	0.9	191
Bavarians:		
Cappuccino, 1/6 whole, 72g	16.6	252
Chocolate, 1/8 whole, 75g	18.8	261
Lemon, 1/6 whole, 72g	13.0	214
Butter Cakes, 1/6 whole:		
Apple Crumble Tea Cake, 63g	6.9	200
Apricot Crumble Tea Cake, 58g	6.4	191
Banana, 58g	7.5	185
Carrot, 58g	12.2	209
Chocolate, 58g	8.7	200
Cheese Cakes:		
Blueberry, 1/6 whole, 75g	13.9	225
French Cream Cheese, 1/8 whole, 75g	17.3	238
Original, 1/6 whole, 83g	16.7	268
Peach Mango, 1/6 whole, 75g	13.9	217
Strawberry, 1/6 whole, 75g	13.9	220
Tropical, 1/6 whole, 75g	13.9	216
Croissants, 50g each	8.5	160

VARIOUS BRANDS - PACKET, FRESH & FROZEN	FAT(g)	CALS
SARA LEE continued...		
Danish Pastries, 1/6 whole:		
Apple, 67g	8.0	195
Apricot, 67g	7.9	182
Blueberry, 67g	8.2	189
Continental Cherry, 67g	11.2	213
Custard Danish, 67g	11.3	207
Pecan, 1/8 whole, 44g	8.8	166
Gateaux:		
Black Forest Cake, 1/6 whole, 83g	14.1	244
Choc. on Choc., 1/8 whole, 100g	27.0	376
Double Chocolate, 1/6 whole, 83g	15.8	275
Strawberry, 1/8 whole, 113g	20.3	324
Swiss Cream, 1/10 whole, 125g	30.0	413
Muffins, 75g each:		
Blueberry	9.8	265
Oatbran	7.5	205
Pies, 1/6 whole:		
Apple Cake, 88g	13.5	283
Apricot Cake, 88g	13.5	286
Berry Cherry Cake, 88g	15.1	288
Traditional Apple, 100g	11.3	305
HiPies, 1/8 whole, 100g: Apple	13.0	252
Blackberry & Apple	24.0	337
HiPies Mini, each: Apple, 150g	24.0	431
Apple/Berry, 150g	24.0	438
Pound Cakes, 1/8 whole:		
All purpose, 38g	8.4	144
Chocolate, 38g	7.6	144
Sultana, 44g	5.7	163
Snack Cakes, Chocolate, 56g each	7.3	182
SUSAN DAY		
Fresh packaged cakes:		
Banana Cream Slice, each slice	4.1	100
Fairy Cakes: Sultana, 28g each	3.6	104
Wholemeal, 28g each	3.9	99
Jam, 28g each	4.1	104
French Tea Cake, 1/10 whole, 35g	5.6	127
Golden Sponge, 1/12 whole, 34g	1.7	101
Lemon Butter Cookies, 12.5g each	3.7	64

CAKES & DESSERTS

VARIOUS BRANDS - PACKET, FRESH & FROZEN	FAT(g)	CALS
SUSAN DAY continued...		
Lamingtons, 58g each	6.0	195
Lamington Fingers (no jam), 20g each	2.5	74
Madeira: Plain, 1/10 whole, 35g	5.1	122
Chocolate, Iced, 1/10 whole, 40g	5.2	142
Orange, Iced, 1/10 whole, 40g	5.4	143
Muffins: Apple & Spice, 75g each	18.5	296
Apple & Spice Mini, 22g each	5.4	87
Blueberry, 75g each	18.8	310
Blueberry Mini, 22g each	5.5	91
Sultana & Oatbran, 75g each	18.2	331
Sultana & Oatbran Mini, 22g each	5.3	97
Passionfruit Cream Slice, each slice	4.1	100
Rainbow Layer Cake, 1/10 whole, 38g	5.7	139
Raspberry Jam Butter Cookies, each	3.6	63
Rollettes: Chocolate, 42g each	9.7	172
French, 42g each	5.7	149
Jam, 42g each	1.9	129
Sponge Roll with Jam, 1/10 whole, 32g	1.6	94
Sponge Roll Chocolate, 1/10 whole, 32g	6.9	123
Sultana Cake, plain, 1/10 whole, 35g	3.6	112
Sultana Cake, iced, 1/10 whole, 35g	4.8	135
TASTEE		
Apple Pie, 75g each	11.3	201
TOP TASTE - MA KELLY'S		
Cinnamon Cake, 1/12 whole, 38g	5.1	135
Chocolate Creme Cups, 44g each approx.	4.5	162
Creme Cups, 44g each approx.	4.5	170
Double Lamington Sponge, 1/12 whole, 42g	6.4	157
Genoa Cake, 1/12 whole, 38g	4.8	136
Golden Sponge, 1/10 whole, 35g	2.0	117
Jam & Cream Sponge, 1/12 whole, 33g	4.4	116
Jam Rollettes, 28g each	0.8	86
Jam Sponge Roll, 1/8 whole, 38g	1.0	116
Lamingtons, Cream filled, 58g each	16.3	255
Lamington Cremes, 50g each	8.5	202
Traditional Lamingtons, 50g each	5.2	184
Madeira: Plain, 1/12 whole, 38g	4.9	133
Iced, 1/12 whole, 38g	5.3	142

CAKES & DESSERTS

VARIOUS BRANDS - PACKET, FRESH & FROZEN		FAT(g)	CALS
TOP TASTE - MA KELLY'S continued...			
Muffins, 75g each:	Blueberry	11.5	262
	Cherry	11.3	250
	Choc. Chip	13.4	289
	Spicy Fruit	9.1	249
Patty Cakes, 31g each approx.		1.8	113
Piece-O-Cake Light Fruit Cake, 1/10 whole, 50g		4.4	165
Rollettes, assorted, 25g each		3.3	100
TRÈS BON Fruit Loaves/Buns			
Apricot/Fruit Loaf average	1 slice, 1/12 whole, 58g	1.7	159
	100g serve	3.0	274
Fruit Buns, average 62.5g each		1.9	171
WEDGWOOD - FOUR-N-TWENTY			
Pies:	Apple Pie, 150g each	16.5	368
	Apricot Pie, 150g each	19.0	400
	Boysenberry Pie, 150g each	16.5	382
	Loganberry Pie, 150g	16.5	382
WHITE WINGS Packet Mixes, made as directed			
Cake Mixes - Country Style:			
Buttercake with Vanilla Frosting, 1/12 whole, 80g		12.4	281
Carrot with Cream Cheese Frosting, 1/12 whole, 80g		14.7	295
Choc. Chip with Milk Choc. Frosting, 1/12 whole, 80g		12.0	278
Chocolate with Chocolate Frosting, 1/12 whole, 80g		14.9	299
Marble with Choc. Fudge Frosting, 1/12 whole, 85g		13.5	292
Cake Mixes - Family Recipe:			
Banana, 1/12 whole, 40g		6.7	145
Carrot, 1/12 whole, 50g		5.0	160
Chocolate Buttercake, 1/12 whole, 50g		8.5	175
Coconut/Banana, 1/12 whole, 50g		5.9	158
Date Loaf, 1/12 whole, 50g		5.5	168
French Tea Cake, 1/6 whole, 50g		5.2	158
Golden Buttercake, 1/12 whole, 50g		7.9	174
Golden Sponge, 1/12 whole, 65g		3.0	196
Madeira, 1/12 whole, 40g		7.0	144
Rich Chocolate, 1/12 whole, 45g		3.9	143
Sixteens, 12.5g each		3.0	58
Sultana Buttercake, 1/12 whole, 50g		7.5	119

CAKES & DESSERTS

VARIOUS BRANDS - PACKET, FRESH & FROZEN	FAT(g)	CALS
WHITE WINGS continued...		
Cake Mixes - Lite Style, 1/12 whole, 50g:		
Chocolate with Icing	3.9	204
Marble with Icing	3.6	202
Muffins, 60g each:		
Apple & Sultana	6.7	202
Banana & Oatbran	7.3	202
Choc. Chip/Cinnamon & Raisin	8.0	215
Dessert Mixes, made as directed:		
Chocolate Mousse, 1/8 whole, 75g	0.2	84
Classic, 1/8 whole:		
Choc. on Choc., 80g	8.5	290
Continental Cheesecake, 80g	15.3	264
Lemon Cheesecake, 80g	12.3	242
Lemon Meringue Pie, 100g	7.3	251
Triple Choc., 90g	15.4	314
Instant Pudding, ¼ whole, 170g, average all flavours	6.0	180
Microwave Moist, self saucing sponge pudding:		
¼ pkt. made up, 150g, average all flavours	20.5	445
Panjacks, 2 pancakes, 60g	5.6	153
Self Saucing Sponge Pudding, ¼ pkt., made up as directed:		
Chocolate, 125g	5.0	260
Other Flavours, 125g	4.0	240
Bakeo, made as directed: Pastry Mix: Regular, 100g	20.0	450
Flaky, 100g	36.7	556
Pikelet Mix, 3 pikelets, 45g	3.7	110
Scone Mix, 1 only, 35g	4.0	116
Fillings, 50g serve: Cheesecake Filling	2.3	100
Lemon Pie	0.2	47
Meringue Topping	0.5	111
JELLIES		
Standard/Sweetened, average all brands:		
Prepared as directed: 1 Sachet (makes 500ml)	0.0	388
1 Serve, ¼ sachet	0.0	97
Aeroplane 'Premium' Natural Crystals: 1 pkt., 500ml.	0.0	315
1 serve, ¼ pkt.	0.0	79
Low Joule: 1 sachet (makes 500ml)	0.0	30
1 serve, ¼ sachet	0.0	8
Jelly Cup **(Yomix)**	0.0	135
Wobblers jelly cups, 125g	0.0	120
Gelatine, dry 1 sachet, 7g	0.0	26

CHEESE & CHEESE PRODUCTS

Most cheeses and related products are quite high in fat. Like milk however, they provide a good source of calcium so do not delete cheese from your diet altogether - simply switch to a lower fat variety or alternatively limit your intake of full fat cheese to small portions only.

TIP: *Devondale 'SEVEN' cheese is a very low fat cheese (only 6.3 grams of fat for every 100grams of cheese - ie. 2.1 grams of fat for every 30 gram serve) that also melts well if you want to use it for cooking.*

NATURAL CHEDDAR CHEESE		**FAT(g)**	**CALS**
Average all brands:	per 30g serve	10.0	120
	per 21g slice	6.9	84

N.B. This includes Matured (Tasty), Semi-Matured, Mild & Vintage (Extra Tasty) Cheddar cheeses.

eg: Allowrie, Bega, Bodalla, Caboolture, Colby, Coon, Crackerbarrel, Devondale, Farmland, Fred Walker, Kraft, Mainland, Mersey Valley, Mil-el, Moo, Nimbin, Norco, Robertson, Tasmanian, Unity/Australian Farmers, Vintage.

NATURAL REDUCED-FAT CHEDDAR		
Block Cheese, 30g serve		
Bega So-Light	7.8	105
Bodalla Light	7.5	104
Coon Light	7.2	102
Cracker Barrel Light	7.2	102
Devondale SEVEN (skim milk cheese)	2.1	58
Devondale Trim'n'Tasty/Trim'n'Mild	7.5	101
Kraft	7.2	98
Mainland Light'n'Natural	8.0	108
Norco Light	6.9	100
Norco Spring Grove	6.6	97
Unity Reduced fat & salt	7.5	101
Pre-Sliced, 21g each slice		
Bega So-Light	3.7	53
Bega Super Slices	5.7	70
Bega Super Slims	2.0	41
Bodalla Light	5.3	73
Coon Light	5.0	70
Mainland Lite Ones	3.2	51

CHEESE & CHEESE PRODUCTS

OTHER CHEESES average 30g serve			**FAT(g)**	**CALS**
Babybel			8.3	107
Blue Brie			13.5	126
Blue Vein			10.0	114
Brie			8.7	101
Camembert			7.9	93
Cheddar			10.0	120
Cheddar Processed			8.3	99
Cheddar Reduced Fat			7.2	97
Cheddar Reduced Salt			10.5	122
Cheedam			8.3	105
Cheshire			9.8	116
Colby			9.6	115
Cottage *(See separate listing Cottage Cheese on Page 59)*				
Cotto			3.3	63
Danish Blue			8.4	97
Edam			8.3	100
Edam Reduced Fat (**Kraft**), 21g slice			4.1	64
Epicure			10.3	123
Farm:	16% fat		5.0	70
	25% fat		8.0	100
Fetta			7.5	90
Fetta Reduced Fat			4.4	70
Fetta Low Salt			10.0	112
Fruit (average) see Fruit Cheeses			6.9	96
Gloucester			10.2	121
Gouda			8.9	110
Gorgonzola			8.9	112
Gruyere			8.9	114
Haloumy			5.1	73
Havarti			11.0	121
Jarlsberg			8.1	107
Jarlsberg Lite			4.8	82
Moo (**Devondale**)			9.0	114
Moo Squares, 21g slice			3.2	51
Lancashire			9.5	112
Leicester			10.0	120
Mozzarella			6.9	93
Mozzarella reduced fat			5.3	86
Neufchatel			8.6	90
Neufchatel Lactos:		Plain	7.4	78
		Chocolate	8.4	115
		Strawberry	8.7	101

CHEESE & CHEESE PRODUCTS

OTHER CHEESES average 30g serve	**FAT(g)**	**CALS**
Nimbin	10.0	119
Norvegia	8.1	106
Parmesan	9.5	127
Parmesan grated 1 Tbsp., 10g	3.2	43
Pecorino	8.1	106
Pepato	9.3	114
Pizza	6.5	93
Provolone	8.4	109
Quark	2.9	40
Quark, ¼ cup, 60g	5.7	80
Quark Low Fat, 30g	0.3	23
Quark Low Fat, ¼ cup, 60g	0.6	46
Raclette	9.0	110
Romano	8.3	112
Ricotta *(See separate listing Ricotta Cheese on Page 60)*		
Ridder	11.4	127
Rosendale	8.7	114
Samsoe	9.9	116
Ski Queen	9.0	139
Soy	8.0	93
Steppen	7.4	96
Stilton	10.5	122
Swiss	8.9	114
Tilsit	8.9	111
CHEESE ALTERNATIVES		
Soy Cheese, eg. **Simply Better:**		
with Chives, 30g	8.1	93
with Black Pepper, 30g	8.3	94
Lo-Chol, 30g	9.5	101
CHEESE SAUCE		
Packet Mix, ½ cup average	2.0	50
Packet Mix, ½ cup made with skim milk	0.5	30
CHEESE SPREADS - CHEESE DIPS		
Spreads: 1 Tbsp. 20g		
Kraft: Cheese Spread	5.0	60
Light Cheese Spread	3.3	48
Cream Cheese Spread	6.8	69
Cream Cheese Spread, Light	4.5	57
Perfect Cheese Ricotta Spread	1.8	25

CHEESE & CHEESE PRODUCTS

CHEESE SPREADS - CHEESE DIPS continued...	FAT(g)	CALS
Cheese/Dairy Dips: *(also see DIPS page 77)*		
Cream cheese dips, average all types, 1 Tbsp., 20g	4.7	56
Browne's (W.A.) Cracka Dip, 1 Tbsp., 20g:		
French Onion	3.3	37
Malaysian Satay	3.7	43
Spicy Mexican	3.3	37
Tangy Gherkin	3.1	38
Dairy Farmers, 1 Tbsp., 20g: Asparagus & Chicken	3.2	39
Bacon & Tomato	3.7	38
French Onion	3.7	43
Onion & Bacon	3.8	43
Mexican Taco/Seafood	3.5	35
Kraft Dips, 1 Tbsp., 20g:		
Barbeque/French Onion/Spicy Mexican Gherkin/Onion & Bacon	4.1	50
Herb & Garlic/Mild Pepper	4.5	58

COTTAGE CHEESE	FAT(g)	CALS
Creamed, ave. all types: Plain, 100g	5.4	123
with Fruit, 100g	4.2	107
with Gherkin, 100g	4.8	108
with onion & chives, 100g	2.3	92
Creamed, Low Fat, average all varieties, 100g	2.0	100
Cottage Cheese, low fat: Plain, 100g	1.0	90
with fruit/gherkin etc. 100g	2.0	85
Jalna: Skim Milk Cottage Cheese, 20g	0.0	20
Slicing Creamed Cottage Cheese, 20g	1.0	24
Dairy Farmers: Low fat/red. salt cottage cheese, 100g	2.5	93
Natural Creamed Plain, 100g	5.3	107
Natural Creamed Pineapple, 100g	4.1	108
Natural Creamed Gherkin, 100g	4.8	108
Natural Creamed French Onion, 100g	2.3	92
Weight Watchers, 100g	2.5	91

CREAM CHEESE - FRUIT CHEESE	FAT(g)	CALS
Cream cheese with fruit average all types, 30g	6.9	96
Philadelphia: Light 1 Tbsp., 25g	4.0	48
Normal/Soft - 1 Tbsp., 25g	8.5	85
- 1 x 125g packet	42.5	425

CHEESE & CHEESE PRODUCTS

CREAM CHEESE - FRUIT CHEESE continued...			FAT(g)	CALS
Riviana:	**Fruit Cheeses,** 30g			
		Nuts & Cognac/Pepper & Cognac	7.0	99
		Poppy Seed	6.5	97
	Pepper Roll, 30g		9.5	84
	Swirle, 30g			
		Pepper	9.5	100
		All other flavours, average	10.0	104

PROCESSED CHEESES

		FAT(g)	CALS
Cheesesticks, 20g each		6.0	75
Kraft Portions, each:	Cheddar	5.8	68
	Chive/Swiss Style	5.7	68
	French Onion	6.4	71
	Light Cheese	3.4	50
Kraft Slices, each slice, 21g:	Cheddar	5.6	68
	Deluxe	5.6	68
	Light	3.4	53
	Extra Light	2.0	42
	Singles/Vegemite	4.7	61
Mainland, 30g:	Chives	8.4	100
	Herb & Garlic/ Smoked	8.4	100
	Smoky Ham	8.1	100
	Green Pepper	8.4	100
Moo Squares, each slice, 21g		3.2	51
Riviana Dutch Smoked, 30g		7.5	101
Weight Watchers, each slice, 21g		3.1	50
Western Star, 'Life Be In It' reduced fat, 30g		3.2	61

RICOTTA

		FAT(g)	CALS
Average all Brands, 100g:	Regular	11.0	147
	Reduced Fat	8.3	130
	Low Fat	4.6	110
Perfect Cheese Ricotta Spread, 30g		2.7	38

CHOCOLATE & CONFECTIONERY

CHOCOLATE

Chocolate is high in fat and calories - no one has yet produced a low fat chocolate! Keep your servings small when you must indulge.

TIP: *When you do indulge in the occasional chocolate bar, try to buy one with a sugar/jelly based centre rather than a full chocolate or nutty centre (this will minimise the fat content to some degree). eg. Cadbury's Turkish Delight has only 5.2 grams of fat and 214 calories. Chocolate coated marshmallow is also a low fat choice.*

Block Chocolate, average all brands	**FAT(g)**	**CALS**
Dark Chocolate, Plain: 100g	28.5	525
30g (5-6 squares)	8.4	158
Small block, 50g	14.3	263
Large Family Block, 250g	71.5	1313
Dark Chocolate, Cream Filled (Peppermint, Caramel, Strawberry etc.):		
100g	25.8	488
30g (4-5 squares)	7.7	146
Small block, 50g	12.9	244
Large Family Block, 250g	64.5	1220
Dark Chocolate, Fruit/Nuts: 100g	30.6	520
30g (5-6 squares)	9.2	156
Small block, 50g	15.3	260
Large Family Block, 250g	76.5	1300
Milk Chocolate, Plain: 100g	27.4	525
30g (5-6 squares)	8.2	158
Small block, 50g	13.7	263
Large Family Block, 250g	68.5	1313
Milk Chocolate, Cream Filled: 100g	24.7	488
30g (4-5 squares)	7.4	146
Small block, 50g	12.4	244
Large Family Block, 250g	61.8	1220
Milk Chocolate, Fruit/Nuts: 100g	29.5	520
30g (5-6 squares)	8.9	156
Small block, 50g	14.8	260
Large Family Block, 250g	73.8	1300
White Chocolate, Plain: 100g	30.0	525
30g (5-6 squares)	9.0	158
Small block, 50g	15.0	263
Large Family Block, 250g	75.0	1313

CHOCOLATE & CONFECTIONERY

CHOCOLATE	FAT(g)	CALS
Boxed Chocolates: *(also see individual listings/Chocolate bars Popular.)* Average all popular brands (obviously there will be a small variation between different types):		
1 chocolate, approx. 10g	1.8	46
Cappuccino Cups (Cadbury) each	4.2	70
Carob, as for plain milk chocolate, 100g	27.5	525
(also see Health Bars & Confectionery, page 112)		
Chocolate Coated After Dinner Mints:		
Average all brands, each	1.3	42
Red Tulip, each	0.9	32
Chocolate Coated Almonds: 30g (approx. 3-4 nuts)	13.2	170
100g (12-14 nuts)	43.8	568
Chocolate Coated Macadamias: 30g	21.0	220
100g	50.0	210
Chocolate Coated Peanuts: 30g	12.4	168
100g	41.4	560
Chocolate Coated Raisins/Sultanas: 30g	5.1	127
100g	17.2	420
Chocolate Coated Fruit & Nut Mixture: 30g	10.4	163
100g	34.5	542
Chocolate Fudge: 30g	3.7	120
with walnuts, 30g	5.2	130
Chocolate Rum Balls, average each, 15-20g	4.5	65
Chocolate Truffles, each	5.0	90
Cooking Chocolate/Bits/Buds/Melts etc. 100g	27.5	525
Compounded Cooking Chocolate:		
100g milk chocolate	31.5	530
100g dark chocolate	30.2	542
Easter Eggs, for each 100g chocolate	27.5	525

In order to calculate the amount of fat in an Easter Egg you must weigh the Egg (weight in grams) and multiply this weight by 0.275 grams.

In order to calculate the number of calories in an Easter Egg must weigh the Egg (weight in grams) and multiply this weight by 5.25 calories.

For Example: 75g Easter Egg
75 x 0.275 = 20.6 grams of fat
75 x 5.25 = 394 calories

CHOCOLATE & CONFECTIONERY

POPULAR BRAND CHOCOLATE BARS, BLOCKS, CONTINENTAL CHOCOLATES ETC.

Each bar, block, single chocolate, or as stated		FAT(g)	CALS
Aero:	milk chocolate, 30g	8.9	156
	milk chocolate, 50g	14.9	260
	peppermint, 30g	9.6	162
Agro, 20g		6.0	105
Agro 'Cranky Crisp', 20g		5.7	103
Anthon Berg liquer filled bottles, each		3.0	75
Baci, each (approx.)		5.0	85
Bertie Beetle, 10g		2.6	50
Black Cat (Cadbury, boxed), average each chocolate		2.0	45
Blackforest (Cadbury, block), 50g serve		12.2	246
Black Magic (Nestlé, boxed), average each chocolate		1.8	39
Bond Street (Cadbury, boxed), average each chocolate		2.5	48
Bounty,	both flavours, 50g bar	13.2	241
	Fun size, 19g	5.0	92
Brazil Nut (Cadbury, block), 50g serve		18.0	275
Buttons, 30g pkt.		8.2	153
Cabaret (Cadbury, boxed), average each chocolate		1.5	42
Cadbury CHUNKY, each 55g bar:			
	Caramello	12.2	260
	Cashews	17.9	293
	Dairy Milk	16.5	289
	Fruit & Nut	14.5	271
	Hazelnut	19.6	300
	Milky White	18.2	301
	Peppermint	11.8	259
	Roast Almond	18.9	294
	Rocky Road	16.2	284
	Snack	11.8	129
	Swiss Chalet	15.0	295
	Top Deck	18.1	300
Cadbury GOLD, each 100g block:			
	Caramel	42.1	588
	Hazelnut	38.3	559
	Milk Chocolate	42.0	588
Cadbury LITE, each 75g block:			
	Almond Nougat	18.6	278
	Hazelnut	22.0	303
	Milk	20.9	292

CHOCOLATE & CONFECTIONERY

POPULAR BRAND CHOCOLATE BARS, BLOCKS, CONTINENTAL CHOCOLATES ETC.	FAT(g)	CALS
Each bar, block, single chocolate or as stated		
Cadbury POCKET PACKS, each 100g block:		
Caramello	22.2	473
Dairy Milk	30.0	525
Fruit & Nut	26.4	492
Hazelnut	35.6	545
Milky White	33.0	547
Peppermint	21.4	460
Roast Almond	34.4	535
Swiss Chalet	28.1	516
Top Deck	32.9	545
Cameo (Cadbury, boxed), average each chocolate	3.4	53
Cappuccino Cups (Cadbury, boxed), each chocolate	4.2	70
Caramello (Cadbury, block), 50g serve	11.1	237
Caramello Koala, 20g	5.4	100
Caramello Koala Giant size, 40g	10.8	200
Caramello Roll pack, 55g	12.7	263
Caramel Wirls (Alexander's), 100g	27.0	509
Caramilk (Cadbury, block), 50g serve	15.7	266
55g bar	17.3	293
15g mini block	4.7	80
Cashews Bar, 55g	17.9	293
Cherry Ripe, 55g	13.4	245
85g	20.7	378
mini fun size, 20g	4.9	89
Chocolate Almond Bar (Alexander's), 60g	22.2	338
Chocolate Crackle (Cadbury, block), 50g serve	16.0	265
Chocolate Fruit & Nut Bar (Alexander's), 60g	19.8	324
Chocolate Gaiety Bar (Arnott's), 35g	10.6	186
Chocolate Gaiety Peanut Bar (Arnott's), 50g	15.7	268
Chocolate Macadamia Bar (Alexander's), 60g	24.0	342
Chocolate Peanut Bar (Alexander's), 60g	21.9	335
Chocolate Raisins (Alexander's), 50g serve	13.5	244
Chocolate Tim Tam Bar (Arnott's), 45g	12.7	233
Choc. Wirls (Alexander's), 50g serve	14.0	252
Chokito, 55g	17.5	247
Chomp, 30g	6.3	143
Club (Nestlé, block), 50g serve	14.5	264
Coconut Rough (Cadbury, block), 50g serve	19.2	277
Continental (Cadbury, boxed), average each chocolate	2.0	43
Continental Almonds (Alexander's), 50g serve	19.5	270

CHOCOLATE & CONFECTIONERY

POPULAR BRAND CHOCOLATE BARS, BLOCKS, CONTINENTAL CHOCOLATES ETC.

	FAT(g)	CALS
Each bar, block, single chocolate or as stated		
Crisp (Cadbury, block), 50g serve	13.9	258
Crunch (Nestlé), 55g bar	15.2	290
Crunchie, 50g	10.2	242
80g	16.3	388
mini fun size, 20g	4.0	96
Crunchie Nuggets, 40g pkt.	9.7	200
Curly Wurly, 25g	4.7	117
mini fun size, 12g	1.7	42
Dairy Box (Nestlé, boxed), average each chocolate	1.8	45
Dairy Milk (Cadbury, block), 50g serve	15.0	263
bar, 55g	16.5	289
mini block, 15g	4.1	79
Dairy Milk Roll pack, 55g	16.5	289
DARRELL LEA:		
Bo Peep, 50g	0.0	150
Chocolate Almond Nougat Bar, 45g	7.7	177
Chocolate Caramel Snows, 50g	5.5	170
Chocolate Fudge Square, 30g	2.7	106
Chocolate Ginger, 1 piece, approx. 15g	0.7	38
Chocolate Ginger Bar, 55g	12.1	203
Chocolate Log, 45g	14.9	183
Chocolate Peppermint Bar, 40g	2.4	110
Chocolate Walnut Roll, whole roll, 170g	20.4	525
Easter Eggs: Dark Chocolate, 100g	31.0	522
Milk Chocolate, 100g	27.0	506
Fluffy Nougat Easter Egg, per 100g	15.0	386
Liquorice, 50g	1.0	128
Peanut Brittle, 50g	9.0	207
Rocklea Road, 50g	11.0	194
Toasted Marshmallow, 30g	4.5	111
Dipstix, 55g	7.2	232
Drifter, 50g	10.6	235
Droste, per piece 5g	1.6	27
Elegance-Dark (Nestlé, boxed), average each chocolate	1.3	41
Elegance-Milk (Nestlé, boxed), average each chocolate	1.3	42
Energy (Cadbury, block), 50g serve	15.1	258
Favourites - Dark (Cadbury, boxed), average each chocolate	1.7	43
Favourites - Milk (Cadbury, boxed), average each chocolate	1.7	44

CHOCOLATE & CONFECTIONERY

POPULAR BRAND CHOCOLATE BARS, BLOCKS, CONTINENTAL CHOCOLATES ETC.	FAT(g)	CALS
Each bar, block, single chocolate, or as stated		
FAZER CHOCOLATES:		
Blue Milk/Fazerina, 100g	33.0	540
Chap, 100g	23.0	480
Dumle, 100g	21.0	465
Bartender, 100g	8.8	365
Fazermint, 100g	18.0	440
Finlandia Vodka, 100g	8.8	360
Geisha, 100g	35.0	545
Lilac Milk, 100g	32.0	520
Ferrero Rocher, each	5.1	73
Flake, 30g	10.2	163
Snowflake, 35g	11.0	186
Freddo Frog: milk, 20g	6.3	107
milk, giant size, 40g	12.6	214
milk, mini fun size, 12g	3.8	64
milky white, 20g	6.6	109
Milky Top, 20g	6.4	108
Milky top, fun pack size, 12g	3.9	65
Lemon/Raspberry Twin, 40g	9.8	194
Peppermint, 20g	4.7	96
Strawberry, 20g	4.7	96
Rainbow Chip, mini fun size, 12g	4.5	82
Tiny Freddo, each	1.4	24
Fruit Gums, 30g roll	0.0	105
Fruit Jellies (Cadbury, boxed), average each jelly	0.0	33
Fruit Picnic, 50g	11.8	233
Fruit & Nut (Cadbury, block), 50g	13.2	246
Fry's Cream Bars, 45g	7.2	196
Fry's 5 Fruits, 45g	7.1	195
Furry Friends, 15g each	4.5	79
Golden Rough, 20g	6.4	130
GUYLIAN: Anniversary chocolates, each	3.8	58
La Trufflina, each	4.8	73
Seashells, each	4.2	65
Hazelnut (Cadbury, block), 50g serve	17.8	273
Hazelnut Whirls (Cadbury, boxed), average each chocolate	3.7	63
Itty Bitty Bicky Bits, 40g pkt.	10.7	198
Jewels (Alexander's), 50g serve	14.0	257
Just Brazils (Payne's), each chocolate	3.6	50
Just Mints (Payne's), each mint	0.9	34

CHOCOLATE & CONFECTIONERY

POPULAR BRAND CHOCOLATE BARS, BLOCKS, CONTINENTAL CHOCOLATES ETC.

	FAT(g)	CALS
Each bar, block, single chocolate, or as stated		
Kinder Surprise, 20g each egg	6.9	111
Kit Kat: 2 fingers, 20g	5.2	100
4 fingers, 45g	11.7	225
8 fingers, 90g	23.4	450
mini fun size, 17g each	4.4	85
Koala, milk chocolate, 20g	5.5	105
Koala Caramello, 20g	5.4	100
LINDT: Dark Lindor (block), 50g serve	25.0	313
Milk Lindor (block), 50g serve	23.5	310
White Lindor (block), 50g serve	26.5	328
Dark Lindor Balls, each	6.2	78
Milk Lindor Balls, each	5.9	77
White Lindor Balls, each	6.5	81
Chocoletti Mint, block, 50g serve	12.0	235
Creamed Filled blocks:		
Caramel, 50g serve	13.5	248
Cointreau, 50g serve	11.0	240
Cognac, 50g serve	11.0	240
Irish Coffee, 50g serve	11.0	238
Orange, 50g serve	12.5	245
Strawberry, 50g serve	11.5	235
Liquor Cherries (Red Tulip, boxed), average each chocolate	1.8	43
M & M's: Plain, 50g pkt	11.5	244
mini fun size pkt. 15g	3.4	73
Peanut, 50g pkt.	13.5	253
Mallow, choc. coated (Alexander's), 15g	2.8	180
Maltesers: 100g pkt.	23.7	487
45g pkt	10.6	219
mini fun size pkt. 20g	4.7	97
each Malteser	0.5	24
Mars Bar: 60g	10.4	263
80g	13.8	352
snack size, 40g	6.9	176
Mini fun size, 25g	4.3	110
Mars Almond Bar: 50g	12.8	244
Mini fun size, 20g	5.1	97
Marshmallow Bars/Chocolate Coated: 100g	13.5	425
20g pieces	2.7	85
Mickey & Friends, 20g	6.0	104
Milka, 50g	13.8	262

CHOCOLATE & CONFECTIONERY

POPULAR BRAND CHOCOLATE BARS, BLOCKS, CONTINENTAL CHOCOLATES ETC.	FAT(g)	CALS
Each bar, block, single chocolate, or as stated		
Milk & Dark Traditional (Cadbury, boxed), ave. each choc.	3.2	52
Milk Chocolate Bar (Alexander's), 60g	20.1	331
Milk Tray (Cadbury, boxed), average each chocolate	2.4	48
Milky Bar, 55g	17.6	296
Milky Bar White, 15g	4.8	83
Milky Way - Choc. whip bar: 25g	4.2	110
mini fun size, 17g	2.9	77
Milk Way - Milk whip bar: 25g	4.6	112
mini fun size, 17g	3.1	77
Milky White (Cadbury, block), 50g serve	16.5	274
Milky White Farm Friends, 15g	4.9	82
Milo bar, 40g (twin bar pack)	7.8	187
Mint Pattie, 20g	6.4	102
Mon Cheri, each chocolate	4.4	62
Moro, 70g	11.1	308
Moro Energy, 70g	13.0	313
Nudge, 50g	10.9	235
Old Gold (Cadbury, boxed), average each chocolate	2.1	46
Old Jamaica (Cadbury, block), 50g serve	24.3	473
Ovalteenies, 15g	0.4	56
Peanut Brittle (Cadbury, block), 50g serve	14.8	262
Peppermint Chomp, 30g	6.3	145
Peppermint filled (Cadbury, block), 50g serve	10.7	232
Peppermint Crisp, 35g	6.3	164
Peppermint Roll Pack, 55g	12.2	263
Peppermint Truffle, 35g	5.4	148
Perugino, average each chocolate	5.0	75
Picnic: 50g	15.2	256
Mini fun size, 25g	7.6	128
Picnic Fruit, 50g	11.8	232
Pinky, 40g	4.7	162
Plank (Alexander's), 20g	2.8	83
Plum Pudding (Cadbury, block), 50g serve	12.9	245
Pollywaffle, 50g	9.9	234
Premium Dark (Cadbury, block), 50g serve	15.6	256
Quality Street (Nestlé, boxed), average each chocolate	1.6	40
Raffaello, each chocolate	4.0	56
Roast Almond (Cadbury, block), 50g serve	17.2	268
Rockies (Arnott's), 45g	12.5	228
Rocky Road Bar, 55g	16.2	284

CHOCOLATE & CONFECTIONERY

POPULAR BRAND CHOCOLATE BARS, BLOCKS, CONTINENTAL CHOCOLATES ETC.	FAT(g)	CALS
Each bar, block, single chocolate, or as stated		
Rocky Road (Alexander's), 20g	3.2	90
Rocky Road (Cadbury, block), 50g serve	14.8	258
Rolo Bar, 40g approx.	9.2	191
Roses (Cadbury, boxed), average each chocolate	2.1	46
Scorched Peanut Bar, 40g ,estimate only	12.8	190
Scout Bar (Arnott's), 40g	8.2	169
Skittles: 55g	1.6	210
mini fun size, 12.5g	0.4	48
Slab (Cadbury): Fruit & Nut, 55g	16.7	276
Peanut, 55g	22.0	311
Smarties: 50g pkt	7.6	224
25g pkt.	3.8	112
mini fun pack size, 12g	1.8	54
Snack (Cadbury, block), 50g serve	10.8	235
Snickers: 60g	14.0	289
snack size, 40g	9.6	192
mini fun size, 25g	6.0	125
Snowflake, 35g	11.0	186
Sweethearts (Cadbury, boxed), average each chocolate	2.9	69
Swiss Chalet (Cadbury, block), 50g serve	14.0	258
Take 5: 40g	11.7	206
mini fun size, 13g	3.8	67
Tempters, 40g pkt.	9.7	192
Toblerone: Milk, 35g bar	10.6	186
50g bar	15.2	265
100g bar	30.4	530
Toblerone: Dark, 35g bar	11.0	183
50g bar	15.8	261
100g bar	31.5	522
Toblerone: White, 35g bar	10.9	190
50g bar	15.6	272
100g bar	31.1	544
Top Deck (Cadbury, block), 50g serve	16.5	273
Top Deck bar, 55g	18.1	300
Tops, 40g	11.7	205
Tosca, 45g	7.6	182
Turkish Delight, 55g	5.2	214
Twirl: 35g	11.8	191
42g	14.1	229
mini fun size, 15g	5.0	82

CHOCOLATE & CONFECTIONERY

POPULAR BRAND CHOCOLATE BARS, BLOCKS, CONTINENTAL CHOCOLATES ETC.	FAT(g)	CALS
Each bar, block, single chocolate, or as stated		
Twix: 55g	13.5	268
mini fun size, 18g	4.4	87
Violet Crumble: 50g	8.3	228
pieces, 9g each	1.5	41
mini fun size, 20g	3.3	91
Wagon Wheel: 45g	7.4	194
mini, 20g	3.6	89
Wagon Wheel, Caramel, 40g	7.5	174
Whip: 70g	12.3	316
mini whip, 30g	5.2	133
White Knight, 25g	2.7	104
White-Christmas (Cadbury, block), 50g serve	16.0	266
Wispa: 38g	13.0	204
mini fun size, 14g	4.8	75
Wobbly, 35g	10.0	181
Yumbats, 18g caramel filled	4.9	90

Also see Health Bars & Confectionery .... page 112

CHOCOLATE & CONFECTIONERY

CONFECTIONERY

Many confectionery items contain high amounts of sugar (calories) and little or no fat at all. Thus the phrase, have a sweet treat and not a fat treat! Do remember, however, that sweets are high in calories and if you are trying to lose weight then you will need to limit your serving size.

Also available are sugar free candies made with artificial sweeteners.

The figures listed below are an average only - because many companies may make the same product, eg. marshmallows, there will be some variation in the different sizes of each sweet from different manufacturers. Use the figures as a guide only.

All sugar based confectionery (regardless of it's shape eg: babies, cats, snakes, frogs, dinosaurs etc.) has a similar fat and caloric value per 100grams ....

	FAT(g)	CALS
Soft Jellies, 100g	0.0	275
Hard sugar confectionery, 100g	0.0	388
Boiled lollies, 100g	0.0	316
NOVELTY CONFECTIONERY each sweet		
Alphabet Gums	0.0	14
Animal Jellies	0.0	17
Aniseed Rings	0.0	15
Aniseed Rings, Chocolate Coated (Darrell Lea)	1.5	40
Anticol	0.0	15
Autumn Leaves	0.0	11
Bananas	0.0	19
Barley Sugar - Gilseal	0.0	19
Barley Sugar - Havapack	0.0	16
Big Bananas	0.0	78
Big Strap, 50g	0.9	160
Big Twist, 50g	0.9	160
Black Cats	0.0	13
Bright Babies	0.0	13
Bubble Gum	0.0	25
Bullets, Chocolate coated	0.3	8
Buttermenthol	0.0	16
Butterscotch	0.1	17
Barley Sugar	0.0	18
Caramel Budlets	0.6	11
Chewing Gum, 1 stick/pellet, average	0.0	10
Chewing Gum, sugar free, 1 stick/pellet	0.0	3

CHOCOLATE & CONFECTIONERY

NOVELTY CONFECTIONERY each sweet		FAT(g)	CALS
Chews (Pascall):	Chocolate	0.5	17
	Columbines	0.5	17
	Licorice	0.5	17
	Spearmint	0.2	16
Chicos		0.1	12
Choc. Budlets		0.6	10
Chocolate Allsorts		0.5	44
Chocolate Eclairs		1.1	29
Clinkers		0.7	19
Cobras		0.0	21
Coconut Ice, 30g piece		8.8	147
Coconut Quivers		0.9	21
Columbines		0.9	27
Country Mints		0.8	28
Dark Bullets		0.2	8
Double 'D' Sugar Free Fruit Drops		0.0	7
E.S.Mints		0.0	11
Eucol		0.0	3
Fantales		0.9	29
Freckles		0.6	10
Flavoured Milk Bottles		0.0	15
Frisco Jubes		0.0	14
Fruit Bob Bons		0.0	24
Fruit Drops		0.0	19
Fruit Jellies:	small	0.0	18
	large	0.0	35
Fruit Gums		0.0	10
Fruit Pastilles		0.0	10
Fruit Rings		0.0	20
Fruit Tingles		0.0	8
Giant O'Jays, 50g (not each)		8.7	228
Giant Twist, 50g (not each)		0.9	161
Glucojels		0.0	14
Go Lightly Sugar Free:	Caramels	1.0	35
	Hard Candy	0.0	16
	Taffy	0.0	25
Honey Bears		0.0	13
Honey & Eucalyptus		0.0	16
Ice Cream Cones		0.0	22
Irish Moss		0.0	5
Jellies		0.0	19
Jelly Babies		0.0	12

CHOCOLATE & CONFECTIONERY

NOVELTY CONFECTIONERY each sweet	FAT(g)	CALS
Jelly Babies dusted	0.0	14
Jaffas	0.4	12
Jelly Beans, common small size	0.0	8
Jelly Beans, medium size	0.0	13
Jubes	0.0	16
Jungle Snakes	0.0	54
Killer Boas	0.0	444
Killer Crocodiles	0.0	230
Killer Pythons	0.0	150
Kool Chocs	0.2	14
Kool Fruits	<0.1	14
Kool Mints	<0.1	14
Licorice Allsorts, each	0.4	43
Licorice, all shapes, sizes, plain, 100g	1.9	318
Licorice Pieces (Pascall), each	<0.1	8
Licorice Sticks (Pascall), 25g each	0.5	80
Licorice - Milk Bullets (choc. coated), each	0.2	7
Laughs	0.0	17
Marshmallows, all flavours, colours:		
small, 5g	0.0	17
giant	0.0	27
miniature marshmallows, each	0.0	3
Milk Bottles	0.0	15
Milk Budlets	0.6	10
Milk Chocolate Twists, 20g serve (not each)	2.7	81
Milk Chocolate Caramels, each	1.7	33
Minties	0.0	16
Moon Rocks	0.0	11
Mentos	0.0	10
Mint Leaves	0.0	10
Musk Sticks	0.3	50
Orange Sherbies	0.2	20
Party Mix, average each (jellies/jubes - no chocolate)	0.0	16
Pastimes, 10g serve (not each)	2.6	50
Peppermints, all types, average	0.0	10
Pineapples	0.0	14
Racing Cars	0.0	15
Raspberries	0.0	13
Redskin Chews	0.1	19
Redskins Bar	0.4	36
Sewer Rats	0.0	125
Sherbert Cone	0.1	90

CHOCOLATE & CONFECTIONERY

NOVELTY CONFECTIONERY each sweet	FAT(g)	CALS
Snakes	0.0	23
Spiced Berries	0.0	11
Soothers	0.0	18
Spearmint Leaves	0.0	12
State of Origin Jellies: Canetoads	0.0	113
Cockcroaches	0.0	113
Steam Rollers	0.0	8
Strawberries & Cream	0.0	15
Strawberry Malts	0.0	19
Sweet'n'Sour	0.0	19
Tarantulas	0.0	148
Tarzan Tubes	0.0	7
Tennis Racquets (Grand Slam)	0.0	13
Throaties Gums	0.0	6
Tic Tacs, each	0.0	1
Toasted Marshmallows	0.9	25
Toffee Chocs	<0.1	20
Toffees, average all types small	0.5	25
Toffee Fudge, 25g piece	3.8	110
Tongues	0.0	99
Tropical Fish	0.0	13
Turkish Delight - plain, all flavours, 1 cube	0.0	59
Turkish Delight with coconut & nuts	2.0	78
Wiggley Witchety	0.0	12
Wildberries	0.0	13
Wine Gums	0.0	10
Wristwatches	0.0	72
XXX Mints	0.0	10

COOKING - BAKING PRODUCTS

	FAT(g)	CALS
Abundant Earth, Brown rice baking mix, 100g	4.5	335
Arrowroot, 1 Tbsp., 10g	0.0	35
Baking Powder, 1 Tbsp., 10g	0.0	12
Baking Soda, 1 Tbsp., 10g	0.0	0
BiCarb. Soda, 1 Tbsp., 10g	0.0	0
Butter/Margarine, ¼ cup, 62.5g	50.0	450
Cake Decorations:		
Choc. Flavoured Hail, 1 Tbsp., 5g	0.5	22
100's & 1,000's, 1 Tbsp., 5g	0.5	18
Carob Powder, 1 Tbsp., 8g	0.0	30
Carob/Carob bits: 30g	8.3	155
½ cup, 77g	21.3	400
Chocolate, Cooking: 30g	9.0	160
Choc. Bits ½ cup, 77g	21.3	400
Cocoa Powder: 1 Tbsp., 8g	1.1	25
½ cup, 50g	7.0	152
Coconut, dessicated: 1 Tbsp., 10g	6.5	62
½ cup, 38g	24.4	240
Coconut Cream, ¼ cup, 62.5g	12.7	130
Cornflour, 1 Tbsp., 10g	0.0	38
Cream, Whipped, average serve ¼ cup, 40g	14.0	140
Cream of Tartar, 1 Tbsp., 10g	0.0	20
Custard Powder, 1 Tbsp., 10g	0.1	37
Dried Fruit, mixed ½ cup, 70g	<1.0	165
(also see page 102)		
Essences/Flavour Extracts: 1 tsp.		
Lemon/Peppermint: pure	0.0	25
imitation	0.0	15
Vanilla: pure	0.0	10
imitation	0.0	3
Other Flavours average	0.0	18
Frosting (Betty Crocker):		
Creamy Deluxe Dark Dutch Fudge, 1 Tbsp., 17g	3.5	80
Creamy Deluxe Milk Chocolate, 1 Tbsp., 17g	3.0	80
Creamy Deluxe Vanilla, 1 Tbsp., 17g	2.5	70
Fruit Mince, ¼ cup, 75g	0.5	200
Gelatine, dry, 1 sachet, 7g	0.0	26
Glacé Fruit, average all types, 100g	0.0	250
glacé cherries, 6, 30g	0.0	76
Icing/Frosting:		
made with butter/margarine, 1 Tbsp., 20g	8.0	100
made with no fat, 1 Tbsp., 20g	0.0	75

COOKING - BAKING PRODUCTS

	FAT(g)	CALS
Icing Sugar, ¼ cup, 40g	0.0	158
Marzipan, 30g	4.5	122
Mixed Peel, 1 Tbsp.	0.0	26
Nuts: *(see Page 167)*		
Poppy Seeds: 1 Tbsp., 10g	4.5	45
½ cup, 75g	33.0	338
Sesame Seeds, 1 Tbsp., 13g	7.2	77
Spices/Herbs *(see Page 212)* average, 1 tsp.	<0.1	10
Sugar, *(see Page 213)* average all types, 1 cup	0.0	906
Sunflower Seeds, 1 Tbsp., 16g	8.2	89
Wheat Free/Gluten Free: Country Harvest,		
Baking Mix, 100g	3.9	367
Bread Mix, 100g	1.0	217
Whey: sweet, dried, 30g	0.3	106
sweet, fluid, 1 cup	0.3	17
Yeast: Dry, 1 sachet, 7g	0.4	16
Compressed, 100g	2.0	93

DIPS

Remember that the amounts listed below are for one tablespoon of dip only. Usually when eating dips you would consume much more than just one tablespoon!

Average all Brands, 1 Tbsp., 20g		**FAT(g)**	**CALS**
(Includes Black Swan, Chris' Home Style Greek, Fresh Gourmet, Poseidon)			
	Avocado	6.3	64
	Caviar	7.4	77
	Caviar (Chris' Home Style)	3.0	46
	Eggplant	2.9	40
	Hommus	2.5	60
	Mexican	6.0	64
	Salmon	6.0	60
	Spicy Capsicum	4.5	58
	Spring Onion	5.5	56
	Tzatziki (cucumber, yoghurt & garlic)	1.6	23
Cheese/Dairy Dips *(see Cheese Dips, page 59)*			
Guacamole, ¼ cup,		24.0	250
Lawry's Dip Mixes, per packet (dry ingredients only - add any extras such as cream cheese etc.)			
	Avocado	0.2	48
	Bacon & Onion	0.9	55
	French Onion	0.3	55
	Green Onion	0.2	57
	Seafood	0.3	45
Masterfoods Salsa Chip'n'Dip, 1 Tbsp., 20g:			
	Chilli	0.5	9
	French Onion	10.1	102
	Garlic & Herb	11.7	113
	Gherkin	9.3	95
	Mild	0.5	8
	Spicy	0.5	8
Old El Paso, 1 Tbsp., 20g:			
	Bean & Tomato Salsa Dip	<0.1	17
	Chunky Tomato Salsa Dip	<0.1	8

DRINKS - ALCOHOLIC

Most alcoholic drinks contain no fat at all but are high in calories (non nutritional calories!) so you can still enjoy a drink or two if you are restricting your fat intake. But remember, the calories will add up very quickly. Moderation is still the best policy!

BEER	FAT(g)	CALS
Ale, Bitter, Draught, Regular, (4.6% - 4.9% alcohol)		
Average all types, 100ml	0.0	36
1 glass, 200ml. (7 oz.)	0.0	72
1 middie, 285ml. (10 oz.)	0.0	103
1 schooner, 450ml. (17 oz.)	0.0	162
1 stubbie/l can 375ml.	0.0	135
1 large bottle, 750ml.	0.0	270
Lager, Average all types) 100ml.	0.0	37
1 glass, 200ml. (7 oz.)	0.0	74
1 middie, 285ml. (10 oz.)	0.0	106
1 schooner, 450ml. (17 oz.)	0.0	167
1 stubbie/1 can 375ml.	0.0	139
1 large bottle, 750ml.	0.0	278
Light Beer		
Low Alcohol, (0.7% 1.0% alcohol)		
Average all types, 100ml.	0.0	10
1 glass, 200ml. (7 oz.)	0.0	20
1 middie, 285ml. (10 oz.)	0.0	29
1 schooner, 450ml. (17 oz.)	0.0	45
1 stubbie/1 can, 375ml.	0.0	38
1 large bottle, 750ml.	0.0	75
Reduced Alcohol, (2% - 3.5% alcohol): 100ml.	0.0	25
1 glass, 200ml. (7 oz.)	0.0	50
1 middie, 285ml. (10 oz.)	0.0	72
1 schooner, 450ml. (17 oz.)	0.0	113
1 stubbie/l can, 375ml.	0.0	94
1 large bottle, 750ml.	0.0	188
Shandie: Beer/Lemonade equal parts, 1 glass 200ml.	0.0	64
with low joule lemonade	0.0	33
Stout, Average all types: 1 glass, 200ml. (7 oz.)	0.0	110
1 middie, 285ml. (10 oz.)	0.0	157

DRINKS - ALCOHOLIC

COCKTAILS **FAT(g) CALS**

Most cocktails have no fat (like the spirits that they are made from), however any cocktail that includes cream will of course be high in fat!

Figures below are an estimation only and will obviously vary from bar to bar, both in mix and size.

COCKTAILS	FAT(g)	CALS
Bacardi Cocktail	0.0	130
Black Russian with Coke	0.0	180
Black Velvet	0.0	180
Bloody Mary	<0.1	130
Blue Lady	0.0	135
Blue Lagoon	0.0	240
Brandy Alexander	11.0	250
Brandy Crusta	0.0	140
Brandy Fizz	0.0	125
Champagne Cocktail	0.0	135
Chi-Chi	18.0	300
Daiquiri	0.0	100
Gibson	0.0	180
Gimlet	0.0	170
Gin Fizz	0.0	125
Gin Sling	0.0	83
Golden Dream	8.0	225
Grasshopper	11.0	280
Harvey Wallbanger	0.2	190
Mai Tai	0.0	245
Manhattan	0.0	190
Margarita	0.0	120
Martini	0.0	140
Pimms	0.0	165
Pina Colada	18.0	300
Rusty Nail	0.0	155
Screwdriver	0.2	150
Singapore Sling	0.0	110
Stinger	0.0	140
Strawberry Blonde	20.0	350
Tia Maria/Kahlua & milk	4.0	160
Tom Collins	0.0	170
Whisky Sour	0.0	145
White Lady	0.0	120

DRINKS - ALCOHOLIC

COCKTAILS	FAT(g)	CALS
U.D.L. pre-mixed canned drinks, each 375ml. can		
Bourbon & Cola	0.0	244
Brandy & Dry, Ginger	0.0	217
Brandy Lime & Soda	0.0	226
Bundaberg & Cola	0.0	263
Bundaberg & Cola OP	0.0	282
El Toro Margarita	0.0	260
Gin & Bitter Lemon	0.0	260
Gin & Tonic	0.0	234
Haig & Cola	0.0	260
Haig Extra	0.0	285
Haig & Dry Ginger	0.0	214
Melon Liquer & Lemonade	0.0	313
Ouzo & Cola	0.0	262
Rebel Yell & Cola	0.0	288
Rum & Cola	0.0	262
Sambucca & Cola	0.0	264
Scotch & Cola	0.0	262
Vodka, Lemon, Lime & Soda	0.0	260
Vodka & Orange	0.0	264
Vodka & Passionfruit	0.0	264

SPIRITS

	FAT(g)	CALS
Including Brandy, Bourbon, Gin, Pernod, Rum, Scotch, Tequila, Vodka etc.		
½ nip, 15ml.	0.0	31
1 nip, 30ml.	0.0	62
Aperitifs, including Campari, Pimms, average:		
1 nip, 30ml.	0.0	70

WINE, CIDER, LIQUERS, CHAMPAGNE

	FAT(g)	CALS
Champagne: Average, 1 glass	0.0	100
with orange (½ each)	0.1	75
Champagne Coolers, 1 bottle, 250ml.	0.0	140
'Champers & Orange' 5.5% alc., 150ml.	0.0	82
non alcoholic, 1 glass, 150ml.	0.0	60
Cider: DRY average 1 glass, 200ml.	0.0	73
average 1 bottle, 375ml.	0.0	136
SWEET/NON ALCOHOLIC 200ml.	0.0	85
1 bottle, 375ml.	0.0	160
VINTAGE: 1 glass, 200ml.	0.0	200
1 bottle, 375ml.	0.0	378

DRINKS - ALCOHOLIC

WINE, CIDER, LIQUERS, CHAMPAGNE	FAT(g)	CALS
Liquers, average all types, 1 liquer glass, 30ml.	0.0	90
Liquer Coffees, average each:		
Cointreau, Kahlua, Tia Maria etc. with cream	14.0	240
Irish Coffee (whisky) with cream	14.0	240
Wine: Red Wines: (incl. burgundy, claret, chianti, shiraz, cabernet etc.)		
1 wine glass, 150ml.	0.0	100
1 bottle, 750ml.	0.0	500
Rosé: still, 1 wine glass, 150ml.	0.0	100
sparkling rosé/red, 1 glass, 150ml.	0.0	115
White Wines:		
Dry (Chablis, Hock), 1 glass, 150ml.	0.0	95
Medium Dry (Reisling), 1 glass, 150ml.	0.0	105
Sparkling (Mardi Gras, Rhinegold), 150ml.	0.0	120
Sweet (Moselle, Sauterne), 1 glass, 150ml.	0.0	110
White: Reduced Alcohol (6%)		
Reisling, 150ml.	0.0	60
Chardonnay, 150ml	0.0	56
Dessert/Fortified Wines:		
Madeira, 1 small glass, 60ml.	0.0	85
Marsala, 1 glass, 60ml.	0.0	110
Port, 1 glass, 60ml.	0.0	90
Sherry: Dry, 1 glass, 60ml.	0.0	68
Medium Dry, 1 glass, 60ml.	0.0	72
Sweet/Cream, 1 glass, 60ml.	0.0	85
Stone's Green Ginger, 1 glass, 60ml.	0.0	95
Vermouth (Cinzano): Dry, 60ml.	0.0	70
Sweet, 60ml.	0.0	90

WINE COOLERS		
Average all brands: 1 glass, 150ml.	0.0	81
1 bottle, 250ml.	0.0	135
1 bottle, 375ml.	0.0	20

SUNDRIES - NON ALCOHOLIC		
Angostura Bitters, dash (¼ tsp.)	0.0	3
Claytons: Dry/Regular, 1 nip 30ml.	0.0	45
Lemon/Lime & Bitters, 1 glass 200ml.	0.0	90

DRINKS - NON ALCOHOLIC

	FAT(g)	CALS
Bonox: 1 tsp. 5g, mixed with water	0.0	5
Bovril: 1 tsp. 5g, mixed with water	0.0	9
CHOCOLATE		
Hot Chocolate, 2 tsps. mixed with:		
whole milk	10.5	205
reduced fat milk eg. Hi-Lo	8.5	175
skim milk	0.8	125
water + 1 Tbsp. whole milk	1.3	51
N.B. For each tsp. sugar add	0.0	20
COFFEE		
All types incl. instant, ground, decaf, 1 tsp.	0.0	4
Black: 1 cup	0.0	4
Cappuccino, average size 200ml. 50% milk, 50% coffee:		
made with whole milk	3.5	75
made with skim milk	0.0	40
Coffee Mate, whitener, 1 heaped tsp., 5g	1.9	25
Espresso: 1 cup, black	0.0	4
1 cup, white	1.0	16
Liquer/Alcoholic Coffees:		
Average all types including cream topping	14.0	240
Milk Coffee, (ie. made with all milk):		
with 200ml. whole milk	7.8	130
with 200ml. reduced fat milk	3.5	108
with 200ml. skim milk	0.0	69
Pre-Packaged Coffee Mixes		
Jarrah, 1 cup, made as directed:		
Brazil, French, Swiss	2.2	56
Cappuccino	1.1	55
Vienna	2.3	57
Nestlé Coffee & Milk, 2 tsp. powder	1.3	39
Vienna: black with cream, 1 cup	7.0	80
White: 1 cup with 1 Tbsp. whole milk	1.0	16
1 cup with 1 Tbsp. skim milk	0.0	10
N.B. For each level tsp. sugar in any coffee ADD	0.0	20
COFFEE SUBSTITUTES		
Cereal/Chicory beverages (Bambu, Caro, Ecco, Nature's Cuppa etc.)		
Average all types, 1 tsp., 5g	0.0	12

DRINKS - NON ALCOHOLIC

CORDIAL	FAT(g)	CALS
Average all brands, made up to 250ml., diluted using 1 part cordial to 5 parts water (1:5)		
Fruit/Sugar Based: all flavours, 1 glass, 250ml.	0.0	90
undiluted 1 Tbsp., 20ml.	0.0	35
Low Joule/Diet: 1 glass made up, 250ml.	0.0	10
Weight Watchers: all flavours, 1 glass, 250ml.	0.0	6
Ribena Blackcurrant: 1 glass made up, 250ml.	0.0	135
Tetra Pak, 250ml.	0.0	140
Rosehip Syrup: Undiluted 1 Tbsp., 20ml.	0.0	48
Diluted 1:5, 250ml. glass	0.0	148
Diluted 1:5, unsweetened, 250ml.	0.0	50

MILK SHAKES

TIP: When ordering a take away milk shake ask for low fat or skim milk.

	FAT(g)	CALS
Average all flavours, 320ml/340ml:		
Flavouring + whole milk + 1 scoop ice cream	14.0	300
Flavouring + skim milk + 1 scoop ice cream	5.0	220
Thickshakes: average 300ml.	10.0	275

N.B. Also see Take-Away foods, Page 217.

MINERAL WATER	FAT(g)	CALS
Plain/Natural: still mineral water, all brands	0.0	0
Sparkling/Flavoured, average all brands:		
250ml. glass	0.0	115
370/375ml. can or bottle	0.0	165
Diet/Low Joule, average all brands:		
250ml. glass	0.0	5
370/375 ml. can or bottle	0.0	11

POWDERED DRINKS	FAT(g)	CALS
Acta-Vite, 3 tsp., 15g	0.3	50
Alpen Blend, 1 tsp., 5g	0.8	20
Carob Powder, 1 heaped tsp., 5g approx.	0.5	18
Choc Power (Farmland), 3 heaped tsp., 15g	1.5	62
Cocoa Powder, 1 heaped tsp., 5g approx.	0.7	15
Coffee-Mate, whitener, 1 heaped tsp., 5g	1.9	25
Drinking Chocolate, 1 heaped tsp., 5g	0.3	19
Healtheries Carob Drink, 1 tsp., 5g	0.4	18
Horlick's, 1 heaped tsp., 5g	0.2	19

DRINKS - NON ALCOHOLIC

POWDERED DRINKS			FAT(g)	CALS
Jarrah:	**Choc-a-Mint**, 1 sachet 11.5g		1.1	44
	Choc-o-Lait, 1 sachet 11.5g		1.1	44
	Choc-n-Toffee, 1 sachet 11.5g		1.1	44
Malted Milk, 1 heaped tsp. 5g			0.5	21
Milo, both types, 15g (3 tsp.)			1.5	60
Ovaltine, 3 heaped tsp. 15g			0.4	56
Ovaltine Light, 1 sachet, 20g			1.4	80
Quik:	Banana/Strawberry, 2 heaped tsp. 12g		0.0	45
	Chocolate, 2 heaped tsp. 12g		0.4	47
Sustagen:	**Gold,** 3 heaped tsp. 15g		0.2	56
	Hospital, 125ml. prepared as directed		1.0	115
	Instant Pudding, made as directed, 5g serve		10.8	262
	Sport:	Chocolate, 100g dry	1.1	374
		Vanilla, 100g dry	0.6	373
Swiss Miss:				
	Diet Hot Cocoa per sachet		<0.1	20
	Milk Chocolate per sachet		3.0	120
	Milk Chocolate with Marshmallows per sachet		3.0	120
	Rich Chocolate per sachet		1.0	110
	Sugar Free	Milk Chocolate per sachet	<0.1	50
		Milk Chocolate w. Marshmallows	<0.1	50
		Rich Chocolate per sachet	<0.1	50
Weight Watchers, all flavours, 30g powder			<1.0	12

SOFT DRINKS		FAT(g)	CALS
Average all flavours, 250 ml. glass		0.0	110
	375ml. can/bottle	0.0	165
Cola:	250ml. glass	0.0	100
	375ml. can/bottle	0.0	150
Creaming Soda:	250ml. glass	0.0	107
	375ml. can/bottle	0.0	157
Dry Ginger:	250ml. glass	0.0	80
	375ml. can/bottle	0.0	120
Ginger Beer:	250ml. glass	0.0	120
	375ml. can/bottle	0.0	175
Lemon:	250ml. glass	0.0	115
	375ml. can/bottle	0.0	172
Lemonade:	250ml. glass	0.0	107
	375ml. can/bottle	0.0	160
Lime:	250ml. glass	0.0	85
	375ml. can/bottle	0.0	127

DRINKS - NON ALCOHOLIC

SOFT DRINKS		FAT(g)	CALS
Orange:	250ml. glass	0.0	123
	375ml. can/bottle	0.0	183
Passionfruit:	250ml. glass	0.0	112
	375ml. can/bottle	0.0	165
Raspberry:	250ml. glass	0.0	106
	375ml. can/bottle	0.0	158
Sarsaparilla:	250ml. glass	0.0	130
	375ml. can/bottle	0.0	195
Low Joule/Diet Soft Drinks, Average all flavours:			
	250ml. glass	0.0	0
	375ml. can/bottle	0.0	<1

SPORTS - ATHLETIC DRINKS

		FAT(g)	CALS
Cenovis Sport Powder:	Banana, 60g dry	0.2	232
	Chocolate, 60g dry	0.4	231
Ching, (Musashi) 15g serve		0.0	58
Edge Isosport:	500ml. bottle	0.0	134
	1 Tbsp. powder, 20g	0.0	6
Gatorade, 500ml. bottle		0.0	125
Isostar, 250ml. bottle		0.0	68
Lucozade, 300ml. bottle		<0.1	216
Nutra-Life Carboblast, 16g powder		0.0	61
Nutra Sport:	Energy, 30g powder	0.0	121
	Recover, 33g powder	0.0	129
	Restore, 16g powder	0.0	57
Purepower Carbo Charge: 1 sachet		0.0	90
Sportplus:	250ml. glass	0.0	71
	375ml., can/bottle	0.0	114
Staminade:	200ml., made as directed	0.0	65
Sustagen: Gold, 3 heaped tsp., 15g		0.2	56
Sport	- Chocolate, 100g dry	1.1	374
	- Vanilla, 100g dry	0.6	373

TEA

Includes all types - bags, decaffeinated, herbal, iced.

		FAT(g)	CALS
Black:	1 cup, 1 glass	0.0	2
White:	1 cup with 2 tsp. whole milk, no sugar	0.5	9
	1 cup with 2 tsp. skim milk, no sugar	0.0	4
N.B. For each level tsp. sugar add		0.0	20

EGGS

Eggs are a good source of many healthy nutrients, however if you are trying to reduce the fat in your diet then you should limit the number of egg yolks that you eat (the egg white contains no fat!). Also be wary of foods such as quiches that contain a lot of eggs.

TIP: *When cooking at home (eg. muffins) use one of the alternative egg replacer powders such as 'Orgran' in your recipes. If you are making scrambled eggs use either no yolks, or maybe one yolk mixed with several egg whites - tastes almost as good!*

COMMON HEN'S EGGS	**FAT(g)**	**CALS**
Average all types ie. free range, grain fed, normal, etc.		
Boiled/Poached/Raw: 1 medium egg, 55g	5.2	71
1 large egg, 60g	5.7	80
1 extra large egg, 65g	6.0	90
Egg White Only, average all sizes	0.0	12
Egg Yolk Only, average all sizes	5.5	65
Eggs Benedict, (2 eggs)	53.00	700
Fried Eggs:		
2 x 60g eggs with 1 tsp. butter/oil	15.0	200
2 eggs (as above) plus 2 rashers middle bacon	35.0	450
2 eggs (as above) plus 2 rashers middle bacon trimmed of all visible fat ...	25.0	350
Omelettes:		
Plain/Herbs: 1 egg + 1½ Tbsp. milk + 1 tsp. fat	11.0	140
Plain/Herbs: 2 eggs + 3 Tbsp. milk + 1 tsp. fat	18.0	290
(Substitute skim milk and delete fat as for scrambled eggs.)		
Add Fillings as Required:		
Cheese 30g	10.0	120
Low Fat eg. Seven Cheese, 30g	2.1	58
Ham 30g	2.4	42
Poached Eggs:		
2 x 60g eggs	11.4	160
2 x 60g eggs plus 2 rashers middle bacon trimmed of all fat	19.0	296
Quiche Lorraine, 115g serve, average only	25.0	360
Scotch Eggs, each	42.0	475

EGGS

	FAT(g)	CALS
Scrambled Eggs:		
***TIP**: Use skim or low fat milk to cut down fat levels and don't use any butter or margarine - try adding different herbs for flavour.*		
1 x 60g egg + 1½ Tbsp. milk + 1 tsp. fat	11.0	140
1 x 60g egg + 1½ Tbsp. SKIM milk + NO FAT	5.7	90
2 x 60g eggs + 3 Tbsp. milk + 1 tsp. fat	18.0	290
2 x 60g eggs + 3 Tbsp. SKIM milk + NO FAT	11.5	180

EGG DRINKS

		FAT(g)	CALS
Egg nogs:	Browne's (W.A), 300ml ctn	5.4	222
	Jacaranda/Unity, 300ml ctn	10.5	244
	Pauls, 300ml. ctn.	4.8	208
Homemade:	1 egg, 250ml. milk, 1 Tbsp. sugar etc.	16.0	341
	With spirits eg. Brandy, Rum	16.0	400

EGG SUBSTITUTES - FROZEN EGG PRODUCTS

	FAT(g)	CALS
Country Harvest Egg-Like, 1 heaped tsp. = 1 egg	<0.1	9
Just White (Sunny Queen), 1 sachet, 100g	0.0	42
Orgran Egg Replacer powder, 1 tsp. 3g	<0.1	9
Scramblers (low cholesterol), 1 sachet, 100g	9.0	163
Yolk Free (Sunny Queen: egg whites + oil), 1 sachet	11.2	156

FATS

These products are a majaor source of fat in the diet and should be restricted to very small amounts only. Try to eliminate any butter or margarine from your toast or sandwiches. You will get used to the taste! When cooking use only very small amounts of oil or better still use a spray on vegetable spray such as Pure & Simple (one quick spray is sufficient!).

TIP: *Oils are 100% FAT! NO CHOLESTEROL does not mean NO FAT! eg. 100ml. of oil = 100 grams of fat.*

BUTTER - MARGARINE - FAT		**FAT(g)**	**CALS**
Butter: Common, Cultured, Flavoured (Herb/Garlic), salt Reduced, Unsalted	1 tsp., 5g	4.0	36
	1 Tbsp., 20g	16.0	145
Butter Reduced Fat:	1 tsp., 5g	2.0	18
	1 Tbsp., 20g	8.0	72
Western Star:	1 tsp., 5g	3.0	27
Clarified Butter - Ghee, (100% fat):	1 tsp., 5g	5.0	45
	1 Tbsp., 20g	20.0	180
Margarine, all types, average:	1 tsp., 5g	4.0	36
	1 Tbsp., 20g	16.0	145
	½ cup, 125g	100.0	900
Reduced Fat Margarine:			
Becel Diet, 1 tsp., 5g		2.0	18
Era Delight, 1 tsp., 5g		3.2	29
Flora Lite, 1 tsp., 5g		2.5	22
Gold'n'Canola Lifestyle, 1 tsp., 5g		3.0	26
Weight Watchers (whipped), 1 tsp., 3.5g		2.9	26
Soya Margarine, 1 tsp., 5g		4.2	36
Dairy Blends (Butter + Vegetable Oil Blend), 1 tsp., 5g		4.2	37
Reduced Fat Dairy Blend:			
eg: **Devondale Dairy Extra Soft,** 1 tsp., 5g		2.5	22
Copha, (100% fat), 1 Tbsp., 20g		20.0	177
Dripping, (100% fat), 1 Tbsp., 20g		20.0	177
Lard, (100% fat), 1 Tbsp., 20g		20.0	177
Molly McButter, (butter substitute), ½ tsp., 1g		0.0	4
Suet, (100% fat), 1 Tbsp., 20g		20.0	177

FATS

CREAM		FAT(g)	CALS
Regular or Thickened, (35% fat)	1 Tbsp., 20ml	7.3	70
	300ml bottle	110.0	1050
Whipping Cream, (40% fat)			
Unwhipped,	1 Tbsp., 20ml	8.0	75
	300ml bottle	120.0	1095
Whipped,	2 Tbsp.	8.0	75
	¼ cup	14.0	135
N.B. Cream when whipped doubles in size, eg. 1 Tbsp. unwhipped cream = 2 Tbsp. whipped.			
Light, (18% fat):	1 Tbsp., 20ml	3.6	35
	300ml bottle	54.0	525
Extra Light, (12% fat):	1 Tbsp., 20ml	2.4	25
	300ml bottle	36.0	375
Reduced, canned, (25% fat):	1 Tbsp., 20ml.	5.5	54
	100ml.	27.5	275
Scalded/Clotted/Devonshire, average 48-60% fat			
	1 Tbsp., 20ml.	11.0	110
Rich, Pure Cream, (50-55% fat)	1 Tbsp., 20ml.	10.0	105
Aerosol/Pressure Packs, average 20g serve (2 Tbsp.)		6.0	60
Coconut Cream, canned regular	¼ cup, 62.5ml.	12.6	128
Farmland:	¼ cup, 62.5ml.	9.1	93

OILS	FAT(g)	CALS
Vegetable Oils		
All vegetable oils are 100% fat		
1 tsp., 5ml.	5.0	44
1 Tbsp., 20ml.	20.0	175
¼ cup, 62.5ml.	62.5	550
This includes canola, grapeseed, olive, peanut, palm, sesame, soybean, sunflower, safflower, cottonseed, maize, coconut oil.		
Cod Liver, Oil/Fish Oil, 1 Tbsp., 20ml.	20.0	175
Vegetable Oil Sprays: eg. Pure & Simple, 5g	3.8	33
Quick spray, say 'Fats & Figures' twice!	0.5	10

SOUR CREAM:	FAT(g)	CALS
Average all brands, 1 Tbsp., 20g	7.5	70
Sour Lite Cream, Bulla, Dairy Farmers, Unity, 1 Tbsp., 20g	3.7	39
Extra Lite Sour Cream, Weight Watchers, 1 Tbsp., 20g	3.0	33

FISH - FRESH, CANNED, FROZEN

FRESH FISH

Most fish is low in fat, however it is the method of cooking the fish that can add significant amounts of fat and calories.

Listed firstly below is a section outlining different cooking methods and the corresponding fat and calories used by each method. Choose the method that you will be using and then add those corresponding fat and calorie figures to the figures for the raw fish that you have chosen from the following list.

	FAT(g)	CALS
Grilled (no fat), Steamed, Poached	0.0	0
Fried: using 2 tsp. oil	10.5	90
in breadcrumbs/flour, with 2 tsp. oil	10.5	110
Deepfried, in batter	21.0	250
Baked, using minimal fat ie. ½ tsp., no coating	2.5	30

(Above figures are based on a 100-150g piece of fish)

EXAMPLE: Fried Barramundi ....
FAT: 0.8 (fish) + 10.5 (cooking) = 11.3gms fat
CALORIES: 110(fish) + 90(cooking) = 200 calories

Fish - Various Types, raw, 150g serve		
Angel Shark	0.6	165
Barramundi	0.8	110
Blackfish (Luderick)	3.6	158
Blue Eyed Cod	6.0	180
Bream	7.6	186
Carp	6.2	170
Cod	0.6	110
Cod, smoked	1.5	141
Flake	<0.1	157
Flathead	1.6	139
Flounder	1.0	140
Gemfish	9.9	195
Green Eyed Shark	0.9	149
Haddock	0.2	117
Halibut	1.0	130
Herrings (see fish, canned)		
Jewfish	1.1	127
John Dory	1.1	135
Kingfish	1.1	143
Kippers (see fish, canned)		
Leather Jacket (Ocean)	0.8	127
Lemon Sole	1.9	125

FISH - FRESH, CANNED, FROZEN

FRESH FISH	FAT(g)	CALS
Fish - Various Types, raw, 150g serve		
Ling	0.5	105
Mackerel, Pacific	12.5	270
Mirror Dory	0.9	105
Morwong (Sea Bream)	2.0	128
Mullet	8.9	195
Mulloway	3.5	153
Ocean Perch	2.3	125
Pilchards	3.5	158
Redfish	6.6	180
Red Spot Whiting	1.1	120
Salmon, Atlantic, raw	19.5	320
Salmon, smoked, 25g slice	1.2	33
Salmon, see fish, canned		
Sand Whiting	1.1	132
Sardines, see fish, canned		
Sea Bream (Morwong)	2.0	128
Silver Bream	4.6	158
Slimy Mackerel	1.2	150
Smoked Cod	1.5	141
Snapper	1.5	135
Teraglin	1.5	128
Trevally	2.6	158
Trout	3.2	150
Tuna, see fish, canned		
Tuna, fresh	0.8	150
Whiting, Red Spot	1.1	120
Whiting, Sand	1.1	132
Yellowtail	7.2	195

FISH MEALS

Average figures only due to large variations in preparation and amounts of fat used.
Also see Restaurants/Ethnic Cuisine, page 175 & Take-Away Foods, page 215.

	FAT(g)	CALS
Fish & Chips: 1 pce. fish (150g) + large chips (150g)	43.0	740
1 pce. fish (150g) + small chips (90g)	35.0	600
Fish Chowder, average serve	10.0	200
Fish Kedgeree, average serve, 200g	16.0	300
Garlic Prawns, 200g serve	18.0	250
Lobster Mornay, ½ large lobster, 375g	48.0	780
Lobster Thermidor, ½ large lobster, 375g	42.0	690
Prawn Cocktail, 125g	9.0	185

FISH - FRESH, CANNED, FROZEN

SHELLFISH & OTHERS		FAT(g)	CALS
Calamari:			
raw 100g		1.2	78
deep fried, crumbed/battered, 100g, approx. 8-10 rings		9.5	205
Caviar, *see fish, canned*			
Clams, meat only, 4 large/9 small, 100g		2.0	95
Cockles, boiled, 100g		0.5	50
Crab, steamed, 100g		1.0	90
Crayfish, *see Lobster*			
Eel, smoked, 100g		28.0	330
Lobster, cooked, flesh only, 100g		1.0	96
also see Fish Meals			
Moreton Bay Bug, cooked, flesh only, 100g		1.0	95
Mussels, fresh (6), *also see fish, canned*		1.5	80
Octopus, 100g		1.2	78
Oysters:	raw, 6	1.4	43
	fried/battered, 6	11.0	133
	smoked/drained, 5	3.6	63
Prawns:	cooked, peeled, 100g	1.0	100
	weighed with shell (as purchased) 100g	0.5	45
	King Prawns, cooked, 1 only, 20g	0.2	20
	in batter, fried, each	4.0	70
	Prawn Cutlets, each, 25g	3.7	67
Scallops:	steamed, 6, 60g	1.0	60
	battered/fried, 4, 60g	11.0	150
Scampies/Yabbies, in shell, 1, 65g average		0.3	30
Smoked Cod, 100g		1.5	95
Smoked Salmon, 1 slice, 25g		1.2	33
Whitebait, fried, 75g serve		30.0	390

FISH CANNED

When buying canned fish choose the varieties that are packed in either brine, springwater or water rather than those packed in any kind of oil.

The fat and calorie contents of canned fish may vary from time to time due to the location of catch, seasonal variations etc.

Average all brands		FAT(g)	CALS
Anchovies, in oil, drained, 1 fillet, average, 7g		0.5	13
Caviar (Fish Roe):	Red, 1 Tbsp., 19g	2.0	30
	Black, 1 Tbsp., 19g	1.0	20
Clams in Brine, drained, 100g		1.0	52

FISH - FRESH, CANNED, FROZEN

FISH CANNED		FAT(g)	CALS
Average all brands continued...			
Crabmeat in Brine, drained, 100g		0.6	60
Herrings, in Tomato Sauce, 100g		10.5	175
Kipper Fillets in Brine, 100g		9.0	190
Mussels, smoked in oil, 100g can, drained		8.5	126
Oysters, smoked in oil, 100g can, drained		8.0	135
Pilchards, in tomato sauce, 100g		5.5	126
Prawns, drained 100g		1.0	90
Salmon:	Pink, 100g can, drained	6.0	130
	Red, 100g can, drained	10.5	170
	Australian, 100g can, drained	8.5	154
Sardines:	in oil, 100g can, drained	12.5	181
	in Tomato sauce, 100g	11.5	175
Tuna:	in oil, 100g can, drained	11.0	170
	in brine/springwater, 100g can	2.0	100

VARIOUS BRANDS

ALLY		FAT(g)	CALS
Salmon:	Pink, 100g	7.0	155
	105g can (incl. no added salt)	7.4	163
	Red, 100g	8.0	168
	105g can	8.4	176

BRUNSWICK		FAT(g)	CALS
Herrings, in Tomato Sauce, 100g		10.0	190
Kipper Fillets, in Brine, 100g		8.0	150
Sardines, 106g can:	in Tomato/Tobasco Sauce	12.0	190
	in Springwater	12.0	180
	in Springwater, no added salt	12.0	195
	in Lemon Sauce	12.0	180
	in Soya Oil	18.0	220

FARMLAND		FAT(g)	CALS
Salmon:	Australian/no added salt, 100g	10.0	189
	Pink, 100g	5.0	141
	Red, 100g	8.0	162
Tuna:	in Brine, 100g	5.0	146
	in Oil, 100g	14.0	216
	Sandwich in Brine, 100g	5.0	146
	Sandwich in Oil, 100g	16.5	218

FISH - FRESH, CANNED, FROZEN

FISH CANNED	FAT(g)	CALS
GREENSEAS 100g serve		
Australian Salmon Cutlets	12.3	176
Australian Salmon Chunks in Brine	2.3	106
Australian Sandwich Salmon with Tomato, 95g can	2.8	88
Australian Smoked Salmon Chunks	22.7	270
Frelish, 100g	4.5	145
Frelish Patties	7.7	202
Tuna: In Brine/total contents	2.0	88
In Springwater	2.0	88
In Oil - total contents	38.0	404
drained, 100g	15.0	205
Chunk Style/salt reduced	2.0	88
JOHN WEST 100g drained weight		
Anchovies	14.0	226
Crab Meat	0.5	75
Herrings	14.0	193
Kipper Fillets	15.0	220
Mackerel: in Brine	8.0	152
in Green Pepper Sauce	20.0	241
in Horseradish Sauce	21.0	228
in Oil	18.0	249
Smoked Fillets	25.0	298
Mussels, smoked, in oil	11.0	205
Oysters, smoked	14.0	228
Pilchards, in Tomato Sauce	7.0	139
Salmon: Pink, 100g	7.0	155
105gcan	7.4	163
Red, 100g	8.0	168
105gcan	8.4	176
Medium Red, 100g	8.0	167
105g can	8.4	175
Sardines, Scottish: in Tomato Sauce	12.0	182
in Springwater	12.0	196
Tuna: In Brine/Springwater	0.5	114
In Canola Oil	11.0	207
Slices in Oil	4.0	153
Sandwich in Oil	11.0	191
Smoked Slices	5.0	153
And Onion in Oil	8.8	167
Spread, 1 tsp., 5g	0.6	10

FISH - FRESH, CANNED, FROZEN

FISH CANNED		FAT(g)	CALS
KING OSCAR			
Herring Fillets in Tomato Sauce, 100g		15.8	205
Norway Sardines in Oil:	lightly smoked, 100g	33.0	368
	45g tin	13.0	150
PARAMOUNT			
Salmon:	Pink, 105g can	7.4	143
	Red Sockeye, 105g can	10.5	171
Smoked Mussels, 105g can		11.6	233
Smoked Oysters, 105g can		12.6	227
Tuna:	In Brine/Water, 95g can	2.9	102
SAFCOL			
Lunch Pack, each pack		7.9	219
Salmon, 100g drained:			
	Atlantic Salmon/Pink Salmon	6.8	151
	Australian Salmon	11.7	192
	Red Salmon	10.5	185
	Silver Salmon	4.0	128
	Smoked Atlantic Fillets in Oil	8.5	167
Sardines:	In Tomato Sauce, 120g can, drained	2.5	109
	In Vegetable Oil, 120g can, drained	7.2	154
Tuna:	In Brine, ½ 185g can, drained	0.6	79
	Sandwich in Oil, ½ 185g can, drained	10.4	152
	In Canola Oil, ½ 185g can, drained	9.1	152
SEAKIST 100g drained			
Cocktail Prawns		1.0	97
Tuna:	No Added Salt	0.5	114
	Sandwich in Brine	0.6	115
	Sandwich in Oil	11.0	191
	Salad Chunks in Brine	0.5	114
	Salad Chunks in Oil	11.0	207
CANNED FISH SPREADS			
Average all brands, 1 tsp. (incl. **Kraft, John West, Pecks, Masterfoods**)		0.5	9

FISH - FRESH, CANNED, FROZEN

FISH FROZEN			**FAT(g)**	**CALS**

The following figures are for the frozen product only. You need to add extra fat (grams) and calories depending on the cooking method ie:

		FAT(g)	CALS
ADD ON FOR:	**Grilling**	0.0	0
	Pan Frying (1 tsp. oil)	5.0	45
	Deep Frying	10.0	90

(Add these figures on for every 75-100gm. serve)

Average all brands

			FAT(g)	CALS
Fish Cakes:	1 x small (50g)	pan fried	6.5	117
		deep fried	11.5	165
	1 x medium (80g)	pan fried	8.5	186
		deep fried	13.0	235
Fish Cocktail Pieces:	deep fried, each, average 30g		5.0	84
	6 pieces		30.0	500
Fish Fillets, Crumbed, per 70g fillet:				
	Grilled/Oven Baked with no fat		10.0	165
	Fried with 1 tsp. oil		15.0	210
	Deep Fried		20.0	265
Fish Fingers, 25g each:	Grilled		2.5	52
	Pan Fried		4.0	67
Fish Sticks, Plain/Crab Flavoured, average size 30g:				
	Grilled, each		0.3	28
	Pan Fried, each		2.5	55

FISH FROZEN - VARIOUS BRANDS

BIRDS EYE (Frozen product only)

		FAT(g)	CALS
Fillets, 71g each:			
	Deep Sea Dory/Junior Crumbed	10.5	164
	Ocean Blue Grenadier/Southern Blue Whiting	10.5	164
	Oven Bake, Crumbed/Lemon/Tartare/Wholemeal	10.5	163
	Tempura, in Batter	7.0	136
Lite 'n' Healthy:	Cheese, 63g fillet	3.3	92
	Natural/Lemon, 63g fillet	4.0	104
	Canola Fish'n'Chips ½ pkt, 250g	12.8	334
Cape Hake Fish Steaks, each, 200g		5.4	186
Smoked Cod Fish Steaks, each, 200g		8.8	202
Fish Fingers, 25g each		2.1	48
Fish Cakes, 50g each		5.6	109
Flavourwave:	Thai Style Fillets, 80g each	1.6	69
	Garlic Butter Fillets, 80g each	1.6	69

FISH - FRESH, CANNED, FROZEN

FISH FROZEN - VARIOUS BRANDS	FAT(g)	CALS
FARMLAND (Frozen product only)		
Curried Prawns, 300g	12.0	339
Crunchy Fish Pie, 300g	18.3	343
Fish Fingers, 25g each	2.3	48
Fish in Parsley Sauce, 200g	9.4	194
Oven Fry: Crumbed Fillets, each	9.2	175
Crumbed Fillets in Lemon, each	8.9	169
FINDUS		
Lean Cuisine Tuna Lasagne, 1 pkt., 275g	10.0	275
I & J (Frozen product only)		
Caravelles, 135g serve: Broccoli/Lemon & Pepper	15.8	265
Ham & Asparagus	17.5	279
Prawn	19.7	297
Fish Fingers: Chunky, 33g each	3.1	64
Standard, 25g each	2.7	68
Tasty, 25g each	2.8	52
Fish in Sauce, 200g serve: Cheese	4.2	145
Lemon	13.0	198
Parsley	5.2	152
Light & Crispy, each fillet, 71g: Crispy Crumbs/Seasoned	6.3	161
Batter	14.6	189
Lemon	11.4	174
Extra Light/Lemon, each 62g fillet	4.5	103
Sea Cakes, 50g each	3.8	83
Sea Shanty's, 37g each	5.0	82
Snack Times, 360g serve: Lemon	43.2	837
Sweet & Sour	43.2	848
NICHIREI (Frozen product only)		
Breaded Prawn Cutlets 25g/30g each	0.7	52
Tempura Prawns 18g/20g each	2.5	42
SEALORD (Frozen product only)		
Dory in Cheddar Crumb, 72g fillet	8.9	209
Dory in Crispy Crumb, 70g fillet	9.5	159
Dory in Lemon Pepper Crumb, 72g fillet	8.4	159
Fish Fillets in Breadcrumbs, 72g fillet	7.2	147
Hoki in Lemon Pepper Crumb, 72g fillet	7.5	150
Hoki in Tempura Batter, 72g fillet	9.8	154
Hoki with Cheddar Cheese, 75g fillet	9.2	160
Hoki with Garlic Butter, 77g fillet	7.4	156
Premium Fish Cakes, 70g each	8.0	158

FLOURS AND GRAINS

			FAT(g)	CALS
Arrowroot, 1 Tbsp., 10g			0.0	35
Barley, Pearl: dry, 2 Tbsp., 30g			0.7	95
boiled, ½ cup, 90g			0.8	98
Brans, *see Breakfast Cereals page 33*				
Buckwheat, raw, 2 Tbsp., 30g			0.7	100
Bulgur (cracked wheat): dry, ½ cup, 75g			1.3	226
boiled, ½ cup, 130g			0.5	115
Carob Flour, 1 Tbsp., 10g			0.0	18
Cornmeal, dry, ½ cup, 85g			2.9	304
Cous Cous, see Sago/Semolina below				
Flours, (weights given will vary with density of flour eg. sifted/unsifted):				
White, Plain/Self Raising:		1 Tbsp., 12.5g	0.1	45
		1 cup, approx. 125g	1.5	440
Wholemeal:		1 cup, 125g	2.5	354
Stoneground:		1 cup, 125g	2.5	356
Buckwheat flour:		1 cup, 125g	2.5	415
Cornflour:		1 Tbsp., 10g	<0.1	38
Gluten Flour:		1 Tbsp., 12g	0.1	48
Instant Success, (**Defiance**):		250g	8.5	845
Lima Bean Flour:		30g	0.4	102
Potato Flour:		100g	0.5	329
Rice Flour:		1 Tbsp., 12.5g	0.2	47
Rye Flour:		½ cup, 65g	1.5	216
Soybean Flour:	full fat,	30g	5.0	126
	low fat,	30g	0.3	97
Millet Meal, ½ cup, 65g			1.8	196
Oat Meal, 30g			2.6	116
Polenta: dry, ½ cup, 85g			1.7	285
cooked,½ cup			0.9	145
Rice, *see page 182*				
Sago/Semolina:	dry, ½ cup, 85g		1.0	280
	cooked, ½ cup, 115g		<0.1	35
Tapioca:	dry, ½ cup, 85g		0.2	300
	cooked, ½ cup, 125g		<0.1	36
Wheatgerm, 1 Tbsp., 6g			0.4	16

FRUIT - FRESH, DRIED, CANNED, FROZEN

FRESH FRUIT	FAT(g)	CALS

Unless stated differently all fruit is weighed with skin & seeds.

TIP: *Not only is most fruit low in calories it is also mostly totally fat free. Eat up!*

	FAT(g)	CALS
Apple, whole, average all varieties:		
1 small, 100g	0.0	48
1 medium, 150g	0.0	72
1 large, 225g	0.0	107
Apricot, whole, 1 medium, 50g	0.0	19
Avocado, average all varieties:		
½ small, 80g flesh	18.0	171
½ medium, 120g flesh	27.0	267
½ large, 150g flesh	34.0	321
Cocktail, 20g	4.5	40
Babaco, raw, peeled, 100g	0.1	19
Balsam Pear, see Bitter Melon		
Banana, all varieties:		
1 small, 110g	<0.1	60
1 medium, 160g	0.1	85
1 large, 220g	0.2	130
Bitter Melon, 100g	0.0	5
Blackberries, 100g (½ punnet)	<0.1	25
Blueberries, 100g (½ punnet)	<0.1	56
Boysenberries, 100g	<0.1	75
Breadfruit, 100g	<0.1	97
Calabesh, see Passionfruit		
Cantaloupe, Rockmelon, 1 slice, 1/8 small, 100g	0.0	20
Carambola, Star Fruit, 5 Corner Fruit, 1 medium, 100g	0.2	56
Cassaba, see Honey Dew Melon		
Cherries: weighed with stone, 10 cherries, 40g	0.1	20
glace, 6, 30g	0.0	76
Chinese Gooseberry, see Kiwi Fruit		
Coconut, fresh, 50g	13.7	140
Crabapple, 1 medium, 60g	0.2	45
Cranberries, 100g (½ punnet)	0.1	49
Cumquats, 1 medium, 20g	0.0	14
Currants, fresh, ¼ cup, 29g	0.1	20
Custard Apple, Cherimoya, 100g	0.6	73
Dates, fresh, 1, 25g	0.0	55
Date Plum, see Persimmon		
Elderberries, 100g	0.3	73
Feijoa, see Guava		

FRUIT - FRESH, DRIED, CANNED, FROZEN

FRESH FRUIT		FAT(g)	CALS
Figs:	fresh, average 50g each	0.1	20
	dried, 5 figs, 75g	0.5	171
	glace, 100g	<0.1	247
Foo-Gwa, see Bitter Melon			
Fruit Salad, fresh, 1 cup, 200g		<0.1	115
Gooseberries, 100g		<0.1	55
Granadilla, see Passionfruit			
Grapefruit, raw, peeled, ½ average, 100g		0.1	27
Grapes:	small bunch, 100g		
	Black	0.1	63
	Black Muscatel	0.1	77
	Cornichon, green	0.1	56
	Green, Sultana	0.1	60
	Waltham Cross	0.1	59
Guava, 1 small, 90g		0.4	22
Haak Tip, see Lychee			
Honeydew Melon, 1 slice, ⅛ small melon, 100g		0.1	30
Indian Fig, see Prickly Pear			
Jackfruit, raw, peeled, 100g		0.3	77
Japanese Medlar, see Loquat			
Japonica, see Quince			
Kakee, Kaki, see Persimmon			
Kiwi Fruit, 1 average, 90g		0.1	43
Kwai May, see Lychee			
Lemon, 1 medium, 100g		0.1	23
Lime, ½ small, 30g		0.0	7
Loganberries, 100g (½ punnet)		0.1	25
Longans, 10, 30g		<0.1	18
Loquats, 1 average, 13g		0.0	3
Lychee, fresh, 1 ave. 15g.		0.0	11
Mandarin, average all varieties, 1 medium, 100g		0.1	35
Mango, raw peeled:	100g	0.2	58
	½ small, peeled, 125g	0.3	71
Marmelos, see Quince			
Melon, (see separate listings) all varieties, 100g		0.1	40
Mellowfruit, see Pepino			
Mulberries, 100g (½ punnet)		0.1	29
Muskmelon, see Honeydew Melon			
Nectarine, average all varieties, 100g		0.1	39
Netted Melon, Nutmeg Melon, see Rockmelon			
No Mai Chee, see Lychee			

FRUIT - FRESH, DRIED, CANNED, FROZEN

FRESH FRUIT	FAT(g)	CALS
Olives, *see Condiments, page 191*		
Oranges, average all varieties: 1 small, 125g	0.1	45
1 medium, 200g	0.1	68
Passionfruit, 1 small, 40g (20g pulp)	0.0	10
Pawpaw/Papaya, peeled, 100g	0.1	29
Peach, average all varieties: 1 medium, 140g	0.1	45
1 large, 220g	0.1	70
Pear, average all varieties: 1 medium, 125g	0.0	54
1 large, 190g	0.0	85
Pepino, 1 average, 140g	<0.1	25
Persimmon, 1 average, 110g	0.1	44
Pineapple, 1 slice peeled, 100g	0.1	40
Plantain, raw, 200g with skin	0.4	158
Plums, all varieties, 1 medium plum, 100g	0.1	34
Pomegranate, 1 medium, 300g	0.2	112
Pomelo, ½ medium, 240g with skin	0.0	45
Prickly Pear, 1, 100g	0.2	30
Prunes, 5 medium, 40g	0.2	70
Quince, 400g with skin	0.5	162
Raspberries, 100g (½ punnet)	0.0	26
Rhubarb, 100g	0.2	18
Rockmelon (Cantaloupe): 1 slice, 1/8 small, 100g	0.1	20
1 cup, chopped, 165g	0.2	36
Sapodilla (Sapota), 1, average 185g	1.3	138
Sharon Fruit (Persimmon), 1, 110g	0.1	49
Star Fruit (Carambola), 1, 100g	0.2	56
Strawberries: 125g (½ punnet)	<0.1	24
each (1 large/2 medium), 18g	0.0	4
Tamarillo (Tree Tomato), 1 medium 80g	0.0	20
Tamarind: 10, 60g	0.0	50
pulp, 1 Tbsp., 15g	0.0	42
Tangelo, 1 medium, 130g	0.0	47
Tangerine, see Manadarin		
Watermelon: 1 slice, 200g	0.2	23
100g flesh only	0.2	23
Wax Jambu, 1 medium, 40g	0.1	8

FRUIT - FRESH, DRIED, CANNED, FROZEN

CRYSTALLISED FRUIT	FAT(g)	CALS
Average all types, 30g	0.0	100
DRIED FRUIT		
Apple Rings, 9-10	0.0	84
Apricots, 6 halves	0.0	68
Banana: 1 only	0.0	105
chips, ¼ cup	0.0	105
Currants, ¼ cup, 30g	0.1	79
Dates, 6, pitted, 50g	0.1	133
Figs, 25g each	0.2	68
Fruit Mince, ¼ cup, 75g	0.4	200
Ginger, crystallised, 30g	0.0	91
Mixed Fruit, average ¼ cup, 75g	0.3	200
Paw Paw, 30g	0.0	107
Peach, 1 slice, 15g	0.0	38
Pear, each ½, 20g	0.0	48
Peel, mixed: 1 Tbsp., 11g	0.0	24
¼ cup, 30g	0.0	65
Pineapple, 1 slice	0.0	90
Prunes: without stone, 4, 30g	0.1	58
stewed, 4 prunes with 2 tsp. sugar	0.1	95
Raisins, 30g, approx. 1 Tbsp.	0.2	87
Sultanas: 2 Tbsp., 30g	0.1	90
School Snack Pack, 40g	0.1	120
FROZEN FRUIT		
Creative Gourmet, 100g: Blueberries	0.0	55
Blackberries	0.0	26
Mango Purée	0.0	40
Raspberries	0.0	26
Strawberries	0.0	20
GLACÉ FRUIT		
Apricots, 30g	0.0	100
Cherries, 30g, 6,	0.0	76
Pineapple Rings, each	0.0	150

FRUIT - FRESH, DRIED, CANNED, FROZEN

FRUIT CANNED	FAT(g)	CALS

Average all brands

The following figures are based on ½ cup (125g) of contents of can, ie. solids and liquids. To calculate the calorie values of the solid contents alone you should deduct the following figures:

		FAT(g)	CALS
DEDUCT:	Per ½ cup in HEAVY SYRUP	0.0	50
	Per ½ cup in LIGHT SYRUP	0.0	30
	Per ½ cup in JUICE (no difference)	0.0	0

Solids & Liquids, ½ Cup

		FAT(g)	CALS
Apple:	Pie Apple	<0.1	55
	Pieces in water	<0.1	45
	Pieces in Syrup	<0.1	84
Apricots:	Apricot Pie	<0.1	45
	in Juice	<0.1	67
	in Light Syrup	<0.1	78
	Nutradiet **(S.P.C.)**	<0.1	36
	Weight Watchers, 6 halves, 100g	<0.1	38
Blackberries in juice		<0.1	50
Black Cherries:	in Juice	<0.1	57
	in Syrup	<0.1	80
Blackcurrants in Juice		<0.1	47
Blueberries **(John West)** in Syrup		<0.1	86
Cherries Red in Syrup		<0.1	83
Fruit Salad/Fruit Cocktail:			
	in Water	<0.1	38
	in Juice **(SPC Lite, Golden Circle)**	<0.1	60
	in Heavy Syrup **(Golden Circle)**	<0.1	103
	Trimfruit **(Letona)**	<0.1	50
	SPC Fruit Cocktail Lite	<0.1	60
	Tropical Fruit Salad **(Goulburn Valley, Ardmona)**	<0.1	65
Grapefruit:	in Juice	<0.1	36
	in Light Syrup	<0.1	76
Grapes **(John West)** in Juice		<0.1	71
Guavas in Juice		<0.1	36
Kiwifruit in Juice		<0.1	58
Loganberries in Juice		<0.1	45
Lychees in Syrup **(John West)**		<0.1	83
Mandarins:	in Juice	<0.1	42
	in Light Syrup	<0.1	65
Mango in Light Syrup **(Golden Circle)**, ½ cup, 150g		<0.1	110

FRUIT - FRESH, DRIED, CANNED, FROZEN

FRUIT CANNED		FAT(g)	CALS
Peaches:	in Water/artificially sweetened	<0.1	31.0
	in Juice (incl. **SPC** Lite)	<0.1	55.0
	Peach Pie	<0.1	35.0
	Gold in Premium Juice **(Goulburn Valley, Ardmona)**	<0.1	78.0
	in Light Syrup/Nectar	<0.1	74.0
	Nutradiet **(SPC)**	<0.1	32.0
	Trimfruit **(Letona)**	<0.1	40.0
	Weight Watchers, ½ cup, 160g	<0.1	48.0
Pears:	in Water/Artificially sweetened	<0.1	35.0
	in Juice	<0.1	60.0
	SPC Lite	<0.1	56.0
	in Light Syrup/Nectar	<0.1	75.0
	Gold in Premium Pear Juice **(Goulburn Valley, Ardmona)**	<0.1	83.0
	Nutradiet **(SPC)**	<0.1	31.0
	Weight Watchers, 2 halves, 170g	<0.1	55.0
Pineapple:	in Juice, unsweetened (pieces, slices, crushed)	<0.1	55.0
	in Heavy Syrup	<0.1	105.0
	thins, 1 slice	<0.1	24.0
Plums:	in Juice	<0.1	83.0
	in Heavy Syrup	<0.1	105.0
Prunes in Heavy Syrup **(Letona)**, ½ cup, 140g		<0.1	153.0
Raspberries:	in Juice	<0.1	32.0
	in Syrup	<0.1	95.0
Rhubarb in Juice		<0.1	30.0
Strawberries:	in Juice	<0.1	45.0
	in Syrup **(John West)**	<0.1	77.0
Two Fruits:	in Water/artificially sweetened	<0.1	32.0
	in Juice	<0.1	63.0
	in Syrup	<0.1	75.0
	SPC Lite	<0.1	55.0
	Nutradiet **(SPC)**	<0.1	32.0
	Weight Watchers, ½ cup, 160g	<0.1	50.0

FRUIT - FRESH, DRIED, CANNED, FROZEN

FRUIT SNACKS		FAT(g)	CALS
Cottees Fruit Snacks, 135g ctn:			
Apple & Peach		0.4	107
Apple & Raspberry		0.7	107
Fruit Salad		0.4	96
Cottees Ice Crushers, average all flavours, 110ml.		<0.1	110
Goulburn Valley Snack Pack, each ctn:			
Apple, all flavours		0.1	74
Apricots/Fruit Salad/2 Fruits		0.1	77
Peaches in Juice		0.1	75
Pears in Juice		0.1	78
Pear Puree		0.1	67
SPC Snak Pak, 140g ctn:			
Apricots/Pears/Peaches ave:	in Syrup	<0.1	100
	in Pear Juice	<0.1	73
Two Fruits	in Syrup	<0.1	90
	in Pear Juice	<0.1	73
Peaches/Pears	in jelly	<0.1	100
Weight Watchers, 135g ctn:			
Average all varieties		0.1	42

FRUIT JUICES

All fruit juices contain virtually no fat at all and vary in calories due to concentration, added sugar etc.

All brands average	**FAT(g)**	**CALS**
Apple Juice 200ml. glass	0.0	85
Apple/Blackcurrant/Strawberry/Raspberry, 250ml. ctn.	0.0	100
Apple/Mango/Orange/Pineapple/Peach/Lime/Pear:		
250 ml. ctn.	0.0	108
Apricot Juice, 200ml. glass	0.0	110
Blackcurrant Syrup, diluted 1:4	0.0	95
Lemon Juice, 1 Tbsp.	0.0	1
Lime Juice, 1 Tbsp.	0.0	1
Orange Juice, 200ml. glass:		
no added sugar/freshly squeezed	0.0	70
sweetened	0.0	74
Orange & Mango	0.0	75
concentrate, diluted 1:4	0.0	86
Pineapple Juice, unsweetened, 200ml. glass	0.0	92
Prune Juice, 200ml. glass	0.0	126
Tomato Juice, 200ml. glass	0.0	38
V8 Vegetable Juice, 200ml. glass	0.1	42

FRUIT JUICES - VARIOUS BRANDS

BERRI

(Berri, Big-0, Daily Juice Co., Glen Park, Mildura, Mr.Juicy, Nature's Own, Patra, Pure'n'Fresh, Squeeze, Sunjuice, Sunrise, Sunup.)

Pure Juices 250ml. glass		
Apple/Apple no added sugar/Cloudy Apple	0.3	102
Apple & Blackcurrant/& no added sugar	0.3	102
Apple Strawberry	0.1	102
Apple, Pineapple & Mango/& no added sugar	0.5	105
Breakfast Juice	2.0	110
Cocktail Juice	1.0	120
Dark Grape no added sugar	0.8	140
Exotic Juice	0.8	110
Fruit Punch	0.3	96
Grapefruit/& no added sugar	0.8	84
Hawaiian Sunrise	0.3	108
Lemon	0.5	66
Orange	1.3	108
Orange, no added sugar	1.3	93
Orange, Apple & Mango, no added sugar	1.0	96

FRUIT JUICES

FRUIT JUICES - VARIOUS BRANDS	FAT(g)	CALS
BERRI continued...		
Orange & Banana	0.3	102
Orange & Passionfruit/& no added sugar	1.3	93
Orange & Mango	1.3	108
Pineapple/& no added sugar	0.8	105
Pineapple & Orange/& no added sugar	1.0	99
6 Fruits/no added sugar	1.0	120
Tomato	0.7	60
Tomato/ no added sugar	0.8	42
Tropical Juice/& no added sugar	0.8	110
Fruit Juice Drinks (various concentrations of pure juice), **250ml. glass**		
Apple Drink, 25%	<0.1	114
Apple Blackcurrant	<0.1	101
Apple Guava	0.1	105
Apple Peach, 25%	0.3	116
Apple Lime	<0.1	113
Apple Raspberry	<0.1	101
Banana	0.1	102
El Fresco Organic Fruit	0.3	107
Fruit Punch	0.3	96
6 Fruits	0.3	96
Lemon, 25%	0.1	114
Lemon Lime	<0.1	104
Orange, 25%/Orange Fruit Drink	0.3	107
Orange, 35%	0.5	114
Orange Mango	0.3	114
Orange Passionfruit, 25%/Passionfruit	0.3	107
Pineapple Orange/Pineapple Mango/Tropical	0.3	107
Pineapple Crush, 35%	0.5	104
Nectars 250ml. glass		
Apricot	0.1	149
Mango	0.1	114
Peach	1.8	146
Tropical	0.3	152
Cups each carton, 110ml.		
Apple	0.1	45
Orange	0.5	41
Lik Sticks 70ml.		
Average all flavours	<0.1	43

FRUIT JUICES

FRUIT JUICES - VARIOUS BRANDS	FAT(g)	CALS
BROWNE'S (W.A.)		
Bodyline, 200ml.	0.0	17
Fruitful 250ml.:		
Apple/Appleberry/Tropical Fruit	0.0	112
Apple, 25%	<0.1	95
Orange	<0.1	95
CASCADE 375ml can		
Apple Isle Sparkling	<0.1	160
Real Apple Juice	<0.1	202
Blackcurrant, 250ml.	<0.1	120
CUSTER & WILLIAMS 250ml. glass		
Apricot/Mango/Guava/Lemon Lime Crush	<0.1	110
Orange Crush	<0.1	92
ESTREL 200ml. pack		
Apple/Apple & Blackcurrant	<0.1	91
Apple & Mango	0.1	96
Orange	0.6	84
Pineapple	0.2	100
Pineapple & Orange/Tropical	0.2	93
FRUTTI 200ml.		
Apple	<0.1	84
Apple & Apricot	<0.1	89
Grabba Combo	<0.1	86
Hawaiian Punch	<0.1	91
Orange/Orange & Mango	<0.1	75
GOLDEN CIRCLE		
Pure fruit juices:		
Orange, 250ml. glass	0.7	105
Other flavours, average, 250ml glass	<0.1	120
Canned juices 200ml.:		
Apple, unsweetened/Pineapple	<0.1	100
Pineapple, unsweetened	<0.1	88
Fruit Coolers 200ml pack:		
Average all flavours	<0.1	86

FRUIT JUICES

FRUIT JUICES - VARIOUS BRANDS		FAT(g)	CALS
JUST JUICE 250ml.			
	Apple	<0.1	105
	Apple & Apricot/Apple Nectarine/Apple Blackcurrant/Paradise Punch	<0.1	114
	Apple & Mango/Premium Orange	<0.1	118
	Grape	0.1	155
	Orange/Orange & Mango	0.1	96
	Tomato	0.2	54
LETONA 250ml. glass			
	Apricot Nectar	0.1	103
	Peach/Prune Juice	<0.1	150
	Tomato Juice	0.1	45
ORCHY			
	Orange, no added sugar, 250ml. glass	<0.1	99
PACIFIC ORCHARD 250ml. glass			
	Apple & Blackcurrant	0.2	115
	Granny Smith Apple	0.2	108
	Apricot, Apple & Orange	0.8	139
	Grapefruit	0.2	84
	Orange & Mango	0.2	93
Premium:	Apple	0.2	101
	Orange	0.2	94
	Pineapple	0.2	115
	Tomato	0.2	53
	Tropical	0.2	109
POPPER 250ml. ctn.			
	Apple/Apple & Blackcurrant	<0.1	123
	Orange	<0.1	103
	Orange & Mango	<0.1	106
	Pear & Pineapple & Passionfruit	<0.1	116
	Pine Orange/Tropical	<0.1	110
PRIMA 250ml. ctn./glass			
	Premium Orange, 100% juice	0.1	120
No Added Sugar:	Apple/Orange & Pineapple	<0.1	105
	Apple & Blackcurrant	<0.1	115
	Apple & Peach/ Tropical	0.1	113
	Orange/Orange & Mango	0.1	101

FRUIT JUICES

FRUIT JUICES - VARIOUS BRANDS	FAT(g)	CALS
PRIMA continued...		
Fruit Drinks, 250ml. (25% - 40% juice):		
Mandarin & Peach	<0.1	115
Pineapple	0.2	107
All others, average	<0.1	107
PURE & NATURAL 250ml. glass		
Juices: Apple - All Flavours	0.3	107
Grape	0.3	155
Orange Premium	0.4	122
Orange 100%	0.4	107
Orange Mango	0.4	107
Pineapple - All Flavours	0.3	107
Juice Drinks, Average all flavours, 250ml.	0.2	109
QUELCH 250ml. 100% juice		
Orange, regular	0.5	108
No Added Sugar: Apple	<0.1	120
Apple & Mango	0.1	118
Orange	0.1	94
Fruit Drinks, 300ml. bottle/ctn., average all flavours	<0.1	128
SCHWEPPES 250ml. glass		
Apple/Apple & Blackcurrant	<0.1	121
Apricot Nectar	0.1	123
Orange/Orange & Mango	0.1	103
Pineapple	<0.1	133
Tomato	0.1	66
Tropical	0.1	116
Zapple	<0.1	120
SPRING VALLEY 250ml. glass		
Apple/Apple & Blackcurrant	0.1	110
Apple, Guava & Strawberry	0.5	120
Apple & Raspberry	<0.1	116
Apricot Nectar/Peach Nectar	0.3	119
Grapefruit Juice	0.4	81
Lemon Fruit Drink	0.3	75
Mango & Banana Nectar	0.5	150
Orange/Orange & Mango	0.4	95
Orange & Passionfruit	0.3	113
Peach, Mango & Passionfruit Nectar	0.3	120

FRUIT JUICES

FRUIT JUICES - VARIOUS BRANDS	FAT(g)	CALS
SPRING VALLEY continued...		
Pear Nectar	<0.1	113
Pineapple Juice	0.3	113
Pineapple, Mango & Coconut	2.0	140
Tomato	1.5	60
Tropical	0.3	107
SUNBURST 300ml. bottle		
Apple Juice, no added sugar	<0.1	144
Orange Juice	0.6	129
Orange Juice, no added sugar	0.2	112
Orange & Mango	0.2	143
Pineapple, no added sugar	0.6	140
Fruit Drinks:		
Orange/Orange & Passionfruit	<0.1	126
Orange & Mango/Tropical	<0.1	129
Pine Coconut	1.0	138
Regency Fruit Drinks 150ml. ctn.:		
All flavours, average	<0.1	69
Fruit Ice Products, each:		
Fruit Tubes, all flavours	<0.1	50
Ice Drops, all flavours	0.0	38
Sunny Boy, all flavours	0.0	63
Zooper Doopers	0.0	15
SUNRAYSIA 250ml. glass		
Apple Cranberry/Banana & Honey	<0.1	126
Dark Grape/Organic White Grape	<0.1	147
Honey & Lemon	<0.1	139
Orange	<0.1	95
Prune	<0.1	150
Raisin	<0.1	215
VALENCIO 250ml. glass		
Apple/Apple & Pear (no added sugar)	<0.1	107
Dark Grape Juice	<0.1	147
Four Fruits	<0.1	110
Grapefruit (no added sugar)	<0.1	85
Orange/Orange & Mango (no added sugar	<0.1	93
Pineapple Orange	<0.1	93
Tahitian Punch	<0.1	114
Wake Up Juice	<0.1	110

HEALTH BARS & CONFECTIONERY

It is a good idea to always check the packets of health food snack items - "Healthy" does not always mean low fat. When looking at the listed ingredients remember that they are listed in order of highest to lowest content - so if any type of oil, butter, coconut or eggs etc. are listed near the top then the fat content will probably be fairly high!

BELLIS each bar	**FAT(g)**	**CALS**
Chocolate Apricot Sticks, 20g each	1.9	76
Fruit Bars, 20g size (incl. Apricot, Pineapple, Orange, Strawberry, Wild Berry)	1.0	75
Fruit Bars, 45g size	2.4	165
Fruit Delights: Apricot pieces, 50g (1/3 pkt.)	2.7	183
each piece	0.4	25
Assorted fruit pieces, 50g	2.7	183
each piece	0.4	25
BE NATURAL		
Almond & Coconut Bar, 50g	16.5	274
Apricot & Almond Bar, 50g	16.4	269
Banana & Coconut Bar, 50g	10.8	245
Carob Coated Coconut Crisp, 55g	13.5	277
Carob Coated Sultana Crisp, 55g	4.5	193
Fruit & Nut Delight, 50g	17.1	263
Nut Delight, 50g	18.1	284
Pepita, 50g	17.6	385
Clusters, 60g each: Apricot Yoghurt	13.7	280
Banana Yoghurt	14.0	298
Fruit Salad	13.7	283
CAROB CONFECTIONERY - Average all brands		
Carob Blocks, 100g	30.0	525
Carob Buttons, 100g	30.0	525
Carob Coated Sultanas, Raisins, 100g	18.5	420
Carob Coated Nuts, average all types, 100g	40.0	575
Carob Coated Rice Cakes: 35g each	9.5	170
50g each	14.0	250
CAROBBEAN BARS - RONOCCO, 25g serve, 1/3 bar		
Apricot	10.1	165
Coconut	12.6	178
Fruit & Nut	12.0	174
Mint	8.8	132
Orange/Plain	8.7	131

HEALTH BARS & CONFECTIONERY

	FAT(g)	CALS
EUROPE each bar		
Apricot & Coconut, 50g	7.0	163
Caramel Chew, 30g	4.4	131
Cherry Coconut, 45g	9.1	178
Fruit & Nut Roll/Log, 45g	12.0	210
Fruit Nougat Bar, 45g	3.5	163
Ginger, 40g	3.0	154
Honey Nougat Log: 45g	11.8	220
Mini, 25g	6.6	122
Jupiter Caramel Bar, 30g	4.4	130
Nut Chew, 20g	3.5	92
Raspberry Chew, 20g	3.9	94
Sesame Bar, 45g	9.3	185
Summer Roll, 45g	11.8	218
Tropical Fruit Bar, 45g	5.9	143
GLENNY'S		
Moist & Chewy Bars, 42g each:		
Coconut Almondine	10.0	190
Oatmeal Raisin	3.0	160
Peanut Snack/Sunflower Snack	7.0	180
Sunrise Nutrition Bars, 42g each:		
Bee Pollen Sunrise	8.0	190
Ginseng Sunrise	7.0	160
Spirulina Sunrise	5.0	140
GOLDEN DAYS (HEINZ)		
Apricot Delight: 50g, 1/3 pkt. (150g pkt.)	3.0	178
33g, 1/3 pkt. (100g pkt.)	1.9	118
Apricot Coconut Slice: 50g, 1/3 pkt. (150g pkt.)	4.3	190
Carob Bars, 40g each bar: Apricot, Cherry, Ginger, average	8.7	185
Coconut	14.6	220
GO NATURAL each bar		
Almond & Apricot, 40g	13.1	215
Almond & Coconut, 40g	13.2	219
Banana & Coconut, 40g	8.6	196
Fruit & Nut, 40g	13.7	210
Macadamia & Apricot, 40g	16.4	204
Nut Delight, 40g	14.5	227
Clusters: Apricot/Fruit Salad	8.0	165
Yoghurt, 35g	8.0	165
Carob Macadamia Nut, 45g	23.8	276
Carob Sesame Fruit & Nut, 45g	10.3	225

HEALTH BARS & CONFECTIONIONERY

HOLEX 50g serve (½ block)	FAT(g)	CALS
Hazelnut	18.5	278
Hazelnut & Almond	19.5	285
Milk Chocolate/Dark Chocolate	18.0	275
Peppermint	20.5	289
Strawberry Cream	19.5	285
NANA DIVER'S each slice, approx. 90g		
Apricot Slice	5.5	319
Apricot Topped Slice	12.9	370
Fruit & Nut Slice	14.6	378
Honey & Oat Slice	12.2	364
NATURALLY GOOD		
Apricot Pieces in Carob, 10g each	1.7	41
Banana Pieces in Carob, 10g each	1.5	59
Ginger Pieces in Carob, 10g each	1.6	38
Pineapple Pieces in Carob, 10g each	1.6	45
Carob Coated Rice Cake	14.4	250
Carob Coated Buckwheat Crispbread	7.8	134
POWER BAR		
Average all flavours, each bar, 65g	2.0	225
SUN each bar		
Almond & Honey, 35g	13.3	198
Apricot Bar, 50g	8.4	211
Apricot Treat, 25g	6.5	121
Cashew & Honey, 35g	11.9	192
Cherry Delight, 55g	13.8	258
Cherry Delight Junior, 25g	6.3	118
Chewy Muesli Bar, 25g	4.0	111
Chewy Peanut Bar, 25g	4.1	106
4 All Seasons, 40g	10.4	203
Hazelnut & Honey, 35g	15.1	207
Honey Almond Nougat, 40g	6.4	177
Macadamia & Honey, 35g	18.2	224
Nougat Roll, 40g	11.6	209
Peanut & Honey, 35g	12.6	197
Peanut Pleasure, 40g	8.7	185
Peppermint Nougat Roll, 45g	11.0	221
Sesame Bar, 45g	9.8	208
Sunflower & Nut Bar, 35g	12.4	194

HEALTH BARS & CONFECTIONERY

SUN VALLEY TRUE FRUITS	FAT(g)	CALS
Fruit Bars, 20g each:		
Apple	<0.1	49
Apple & Plum/Apple & Apricot	<0.1	45
Apricot/Peach & Pear	<0.1	41
Pear	<0.1	54
Carob Fruit Bar:		
regular, 50g	14.6	240
no added sugar, 50g	13.7	237
Yoghurt Fruit Bar:		
regular, 50g	13.5	227
no added sugar, 50g	16.4	238
YOGHURT COATED CONFECTIONERY		
Average all brands:		
Yoghurt Buttons, 100g	32.0	520
Yoghurt Coated Sultanas, Raisins, 100g	22.0	450
Yoghurt Coated Apricot Pieces, 100g	32.0	500
Yoghurt Coated Nuts, 100g	44.0	610
Yoghurt Coated Rice Cake, 50g	15.0	260
Yoghurt Clusters, average all flavours:		
Go Natural, 35g	8.2	163
Be Natural, 60g	13.9	290
Z & E BARS each bar		
Date & Walnut, 70g	17.0	327
Fruit & Nut, 70g	18.8	334
Zorans Sunflower, 70g	29.2	396

HEALTH SNACK FOODS - MUESLI BARS

AUSSIE BODIES each slice	**FAT(g)**	**CALS**
Amino Treat Bar	8.0	210
Energy Extender Slice	6.3	318
Trim Energy Slice	2.5	270
Perfect Protein Slice	6.6	315
AUSTRALIA'S CHOICE (K-Mart) Muesli Bars		
Choc Chip, each, 31.3g	5.4	131
Sultana & Almond, each, 31.3g	4.9	131
Tropical Fruit, each, 31.3g	3.9	126
BE NATURAL - GO NATURAL		
Apricot Yoghurt Clusters, each, 35g	8.0	165
60g	13.7	280
Banana Yoghurt Clusters, each, 60g	14.0	298
Fruit Salad Yoghurt Clusters, each, 35g	8.2	165
60g	13.7	283
BERRIMA COOKIE CO.		
Original Muesli, Muesli with Carob/Fruit Chunks average all types, 70-75g each	20.7	420
BODY-LITE GOLD (AMINOACTIVE)		
Each bar, 90g each	2.0	275
CARROBBEAN		
Carob Coated Rice Cake, 30g	8.7	151
ENERGY		
Energy Sports Slice, Carob Coated, 100g	10.2	362
FARMLAND Muesli Bars, 32g each		
Apricot & Coconut	3.8	126
Choc. Chip	4.5	131
3 Fruits	3.6	126
Choc. Coated: Cherry & Coconut	7.8	160
Fruit & Nut	7.7	160
Nut Trio	9.7	170
Peppermint	8.2	162
FLIPPS		
Muesli Bars, each bar, 31.3g		
Apricot/Passion, White Chocolate	4.3	159
Cherry Coconut, Chocolate	5.0	162
Fruit Delight, White Chocolate	4.3	157

HEALTH SNACK FOODS - MUESLI BARS

FLIPPS continued..	**FAT(g)**	**CALS**
Honeycomb/Banana, Chocolate Coated	1.4	147
Orange/Mango	3.4	132
Peach/Apple/Blackcurrant	3.0	125
Peach/Raspberry	2.6	123
Strawberry/Banana	2.5	123
FREEDOM FOODS		
Carob Fruit Cluster, 60g	8.2	234
Carob Rice Cookies, each	2.1	38
Carob Rice Crispbread, each	8.3	128
Mini Carob Rice Cakes, each	2.2	39
Fruit Cookies, each	1.3	74
Yoghurt Slice, 100g	19.4	415
Freedom Energy Slice, 95g	9.7	295
GLENNY'S		
Brown Rice Treats each		
Carob Mint with Oatbran, 49g	1.0	170
Cinnamon & Raisin, 49g	2.0	180
Peanut & Raisin, 56g	5.0	210
Plain & Fancy, 35g	1.0	120
Raisin Bran Treat, 49g	1.0	170
Toasted Almond with Oatbran, 49g	5.0	200
Moist & Chewy Bars each, 42g		
Coconut Almondino	10.0	190
Oatmeal Raisin	3.0	160
Peanut Snack/Sunflower	7.0	180
Fat Free Snack Bars all flavours	<0.5	120
GOLD CREST		
Fruitz Mueli Bars, each bar, 31.3g		
Apricot Passion, Yoghurt Coated	3.9	135
Cherry Coconut, Chocolate Coated	4.7	143
Fruit Salad, Yoghurt Coated	4.0	145
Honeycomb, Chocolate Coated	5.8	136
Muesli Bites, each 'bite', 20g,		
Apricot Passion, Yoghurt Coated	3.6	87
Cherry Coconut, Chocolate Coated	3.8	88
Honeycomb, Chocolate Coated	3.7	87

HEALTH SNACK FOODS - MUESLI BARS

HEATHER BRAE		FAT(g)	CALS
	Honey Crunch Cookie, 70g	18.0	334
	Muesli Crunch Cookie, 70g	28.0	385
HORLEY'S			
	Energiser Sports Bar, 60g	2.1	220
HOUSE OF TREATS			
Aussie Treats:	Apricot & Almond Cookie, 50g	15.0	240
	Carob & Raisin Cookie, 50g	15.0	243
	Anzac Cookie/Anzac Slice, 85g	24.0	413
	Choc. Coated Anzac, 60g	17.0	301
	Choc.Chip Cookie, 85g	20.0	408
	Choc. Chip Round Cake, 85g	21.0	399
	Honey & Oats Treat, 100g	18.0	411
	Natural Muesli Treat, 85g	20.0	374
Tahini Treats:	Apricot & Almond, 85g	27.0	422
	Carob & Sultana, 85g	20.0	408
	Ultimate, 65g	20.0	315
MAGIC APPLE			
Golden Bakes each:	Anzac Biscuit, 90g	19.8	365
	Banana & Pecan, 90g	18.9	359
	Choc. Chip Cookie, 90g	25.7	421
	Cinnamon & Almond, 90g	20.3	353
	Currant & Lemon Crunch, 80g	13.6	304
	Date & Muesli, 140g	23.8	487
Slices each:	Almond Apricot Slice, 70g	14.7	274
	Almond Munchie, 90g	20.3	378
	Boosta Break, 80g	30.0	405
	Choc. Nut Crunch, 80g	17.6	329
	Flap Jack, 90g	17.1	372
MELOATS			
	Banana Yoghurt Coated Bar, 75g	14.6	310
	Carob Coated Bar, 75g	14.6	310
	Original/Apricot/Fruit & Nut Bars, 125g each	23.3	496
MUSASHI each slice			
	Amino Gold, 95g	9.0	300
	Amoni Red diet slice, 95g	9.0	290
	Amino Trim, 95g	9.7	277
	Slim, 95g	4.5	240

HEALTH SNACK FOODS - MUESLI BARS

	FAT(g)	CALS
POWER BAR		
All Flavours, 65g	2.0	225
PUREPOWER		
Energy Bar, 65g	3.0	240
SUNIBRITE		
Round Cakes, each		
Apricot Yoghurt Dipped, 90g	21.2	335
Carob Chip, 90g	15.0	367
Choc Chip, 90g	14.8	366
Date & Walnut, 90g	11.0	298
Farmhouse Fruit Bun, 90g	12.8	324
Oatmeal & Fruit, 90g	11.9	345
Oatmeal & Fruit, Carob Dipped, 90g	14.9	368
Pecan & Sultana, 90g	11.6	306
Raisin & Hazelnut, 90g	11.7	312
Stockade Bun, Caramel Coated, 90g	22.6	411
Yoghurt Coated Fruity Bun, 90g	16.8	353
Slices, each		
Banana & Honey Slice, 75g	13.7	285
Carrot Slice, 75g	14.4	289
Honey & Date Slice, 75g	15.3	306
Muesli Slice, 85g	18.0	374
Muesli Slice, Carob Coated, 85g	18.6	393
Muesli & Apricot Slice, 85g	16.0	361
Muesli & Apricot, Yoghurt Coated, 85g	17.5	359
Orange, Mango & Pecan Slice, 75g	14.0	310
Strawberry Slice, Yoghurt Coated, 85g	17.5	361
ULTRA SLIM		
Oat Bran & Cherry, 40g each	3.9	149
Oat Bran & Apricot, 40g each	3.9	149
UNCLE TOBY'S		
Breakfast Bars each		
Fibreplus	3.0	173
Lite Start	2.3	136
Sports Plus	2.5	145
Clusters, 60g each	9.5	249

HEALTH SNACK FOODS - MUESLI BARS

UNCLE TOBY'S continued...		FAT(g)	CALS
Muesli Bars, 31.3g each			
Chewy:	Apricot & Coconut	3.3	120
	Banana Choc. Chip	4.6	132
	Blackcurrant & Apple	3.5	127
	Choc. Chip	4.8	132
	Fruit Selection	3.1	120
	Peanut Butter	4.2	128
	Peppermint Choc. Chip	4.8	132
	Three Fruits	3.2	119
	Tropical	2.9	120
Crunchy:	Apricot	3.9	126
	Coconut Choc. Chip	4.8	135
	Nut Crumble	6.2	144
Roll-Ups, average all types, each bar		1.0	57
Topform each bar:	Cherry	5.9	173
	Fruit & Nut	5.6	172
	Pineapple	5.5	172
Topps	**Fruit,** All Flavours, each bar	4.5	137
	Yoghurt: Apricot/Strawberry	5.5	138
	Fruit Salad	5.2	137
	Mango & Passionfruit	5.3	135
	Nut Crumble	6.2	144
	Raspberry	5.8	138
Wrapps	each bar, 33.4g		
	Apricot & Coconut	7.4	149
	Capuccino & Hazelnut	8.7	166
	Cherry & Coconut	7.4	147
	Cherry & Coconut, mini, 16.7g	4.4	80
	Honeycomb	7.3	160
	Nut Combo	8.8	159
	Nut Combo, mini, 16.7g	4.4	80
	Peppermint	8.0	155
	Peppermint, mini, 16.7g	4.0	78
VICTORY			
Sports Bar, 50g		2.7	157

ICE CREAM & ICE CONFECTIONS

There is an excellent variety of tasty low fat ice creams and confections available for the wise shopper.

Ice cream volumes are calculated using the common 100ml. size ice cream scoop available in supermarkets & kitchenware stores. The weight in grams of 100ml. of ice cream will vary depending on the creaminess of the ice cream. Most standard ice creams however, will equal 45-50 grams for each 100ml. scoop.

ALL BRANDS - AVERAGE		**FAT(g)**	**CALS**

Again, depending on the creaminess (fat content) of the ice cream, fat & calorie values will vary accordingly.

		FAT(g)	CALS
Extra Low Fat:	eg. **Streets Too Good To Be True,** 1 scoop, 100ml., 48g	0.5	92
Low Fat:	eg. **Peters Light & Creamy,** 1 scoop, 100ml., 49g	1.3	70
Fat Reduced:	eg. **Streets Blue Ribbon Light,** 1 scoop, 100ml., 48g	3.0	73
Standard:	all flavours, 1 scoop, 100ml. 48g	5.0	91
Extra Creamy:	eg. **Browne's Connoisseur,** 1 scoop, 100ml., 70g	10.5	165
Super Creamy:	eg. **Sara Lee, Homer Hudson,** 1 scoop, 100ml., 90g	18.0	265

DIFFERENT ICE CREAMS - CONFECTIONS

		FAT(g)	CALS
Cassata, 1 average serve		15.0	215
Fried Ice Cream Balls, each		13.0	175
Gelato, 2 scoops		0.0	75
Soft Serve, 100ml.		2.5	90
Sorbet:	with milk, 100ml.	3.7	100
	no milk, 100ml.	0.3	55
Tofu:	Standard, 1 scoop, 100ml	5.0	75
	Low Fat, 1 scoop, 100ml.	1.0	60
	Soft Serve, 110g (200ml.)	8.0	190
Theatre Choc Top, 1		10.0	203
Vitari:	100ml.	<0.1	60
	Soft serve with cone, 1	0.0	90
Yoghurt:	Soft Serve - low fat with cone, 100ml.	3.0	105
	Soft Serve - non fat with cone, 100ml.	0.0	80

ICE CREAM & ICE CONFECTIONS

MILK BARS - TAKE AWAY	FAT(g)	CALS
Flavoured ice cream, 100ml. scoop (average all brands)		
Arctic Mint	6.9	134
Banana Split	5.6	107
Boysenberry	4.9	111
Boysenberry Swirl	6.6	133
Butterscotch	7.0	122
Butterscotch Brickle	5.3	112
Cappuccino	6.0	110
Caramel Fudge	7.4	141
Chocolate	6.2	128
Chocolate Choc. Chip	7.6	137
English Toffee	6.0	120
French Vanilla	7.0	122
Fruit Liquer Cream	7.0	130
Honeycomb	7.3	141
Jaffa	6.7	119
Licorice	6.0	86
Macadamia Nut	8.2	129
Mango	6.0	110
Passionfruit Swirl	5.5	112
Peanut Choc.	7.1	127
Peppermint Choc. Chip	6.7	124
Rum & Raisin	5.5	110
Spearmint	8.2	142
Triple Swirl	5.2	97
Vanilla	5.2	98
Vanilla Choc. Chip	7.5	135
Watermelon	7.0	122
Wild Strawberry	6.7	125
Yoghurt, average all flavours	2.0	88
ICE CREAM CONES		
Single	<0.1	16
Double	<0.1	24
Giant, large waffle cone	1.0	80
Wafer	<0.1	8
Betta Cones, all types, each	0.1	15
ICE CREAM TOPPINGS *(also see Page 213)*		
Syrup: Average all flavours 1 Tbsp., 20ml	0.1	45
Low Joule Syrup (**Cottees, Weight Watchers**), 20ml	0.1	5
Ice Magic/Cottees, 1 Tbsp., 20g	10.0	130

ICE CREAM & ICE CONFECTIONS

VARIOUS BRANDS	FAT(g)	CALS
BASKIN ROBBINS 1 scoop		
Chilly Burgers, vanilla, each	11.0	240
Cones: sugar, each	1.0	60
waffle, each	2.0	140
Deluxe: Butter Pecan, Choc. Chip, Choc. Mousse Royale, Cookies'n'Cream, Macadamia Nut'n'Cream, Pralines'n'Cream, Rocky Road, World Class Chocolate...	14.0	280
Vanilla, Passionfruit, Mango & Cream, Rum & Raisin...	14.0	240
Very Berry Strawberry	10.0	220
Frozen Yoghurt, ½ cup	1.0	120
Light: Praline Dream, ½ cup	6.0	130
Strawberry Royal, ½ cup	3.0	110
Sherbert & Ices, 1 scoop: Daiquiri	0.0	140
Orange	2.0	160
Soft Serve Sorbet, ½ cup	0.0	100
BROWNE'S		
Connoisseur Ice Cream, 100ml. scoop		
Chocolate Obsession	12.0	203
New England Butter Pecan	12.2	188
Old English Toffee	12.1	192
Strawberry Romanoff	9.1	174
BULLA		
Ice Cream, 100ml. scoop		
Lite'n'Natural low fat	0.7	58
Soft Serve, 100ml.	5.3	96
Yoghurt Frozen, Plain 100ml. (50g)	2.8	72
Fruit Cups, 100g each	5.4	144
Fruit Sticks, 75g each	4.1	108
CADBURY		
Cherry Ripe, 40g	9.0	153
Crunchie, 55g	11.8	208
Freddo, 55g	7.5	130
Tempo, 55g	11.8	183
CHARIOTO		
Frozen Yoghurt: Low Fat, 100g	2.9	69
Reduced Fat, 100g	6.0	94

CHARIOTO continued...		FAT(g)	CALS
Gourmet Ice Cream, 100ml./50g scoop			
	Chocolate	5.7	95
	Strawberry	5.5	90
	Vanilla	6.0	96
Diet Lite Low Fat Ice Cream, 100ml/50g scoop			
	Chocolate	1.7	47
	Vanilla	1.6	46
Sorbet: 50g (1 slice)		0.0	47
Tofu Gourmet Low Fat: 50g serve:	Chocolate	1.5	74
	Strawberry	1.2	70
	Vanilla	1.4	74
DAIRY BELL 100ml. scoop			
Reduced Fat Vanilla		2.8	77
Dairy Bell Lite, no added sugar		2.1	56
Snow Boy Polyunsaturated		5.0	90
FARMLAND			
Ultimate, 100ml scoop			
	Chocolate with Cherry Swirl	11.0	189
	Old English Toffee with Pecans	12.7	225
	Vanilla Supreme	11.4	177
FRANKLINS - NO FRILLS			
Standard, all flavours, 100ml. scoop		5.0	102
GISÉ			
Crème Glacé Soft Serve, 100ml.		<0.1	21
Frozen Dessert Mix, all flavours, 100g		<0.1	30
GOLD CREST			
Ices, each		<0.1	20
HOMER HUDSON 100ml. scoop, 90-95g			
Butter Pecan		19.0	270
Chocolate Rock		17.2	269
Coffee Almond		18.4	262
Hoboken Crunch		14.6	251
Strawberry		13.0	222
MARS			
Mars, 60ml. bar		11.7	200
Snickers, 60ml. bar		13.9	227

ICE CREAM & ICE CONFECTIONS

NORCO 100ml. scoop, 50g		FAT(g)	CALS
Natural:	Chocolate	5.3	98
	Coffee	5.6	99
	Vanilla	5.3	96
	Vanilla with Mango	5.5	96
	Vanilla with Boysenberry	5.3	102
	Vanilla with Macadamia	7.4	113
	Choc. Coated Macadamia in Vanilla	7.0	225
	Choc. Coated Hokey Pokey in Vanilla	6.4	113
	Chocolate, Choc. Chip & Vanilla	5.4	99
	Tangerine Choc. Chip	5.7	102
Light Low Fat Vanilla		1.9	71
Standard Vanilla		5.0	88
Gold Vanilla		7.0	110
Low Cholesterol Frozen Dessert, 50g		4.8	102
Frozen Fruit Yoghurt, 50g		2.0	67
OAK			
Party Cups, 125ml.		6.5	118
Pleasure Bars		9.0	160
Reduced Fat ice cream, all flavours, 100ml.		3.2	77
PAUL'S & PETER'S Tubs, 100ml. scoop, 50g			
Paul's Standard:	Chocolate	4.9	91
	Neapolitan/Vanilla	4.8	89
	Vanilla Choc. Chip	6.1	104
Paul's Extra Cream:	Butterscotch Brickle	4.9	99
	Double Choc. Chip	5.6	104
	Peppermint	4.9	102
	Vanilla	4.8	90
Peter's Original:	Caramel Swirl/Vanilla	4.9	91
	Chocolate/Neapolitan	5.0	92
	Sundae Twist	4.7	97
	Vanilla Choc. Chip	6.3	106
Natural:	Golden Crunch	7.1	123
	Choc. Caramel Eclair	7.3	124
	Rich Vanilla/Wildberry Swirl	5.6	104
Natural Exotics:	Mocha Almond Fudge	7.2	120
	Strawberries & Cream	5.6	104
	Toffee Macadamia	7.9	127
	Vanilla Francaise	5.9	101
Light & Creamy:	Chocolate Swirl	1.6	73
	Strawberry	1.5	74
	Vanilla	1.5	69

ICE CREAM & ICE CONFECTIONS

PAUL'S & PETER'S Tubs, 100ml. scoop, 50g		FAT(g)	CALS
Light & Creamy Exotics:			
	Butterscotch Crunch	1.8	85
	Classic Strawberry	1.4	74
	Peach Passion	1.4	74
	Rich Mint Chocolate	1.7	78
Peter's Funfoods:	Chunky Choc.Honeycomb	3.8	86
	Cool Bananas	4.6	97
	Crazy Cosmic Swirl	3.2	75
Peter's Carbohydrate Modified		5.3	103

PAUL'S & PETER'S NOVELTY BARS - ICES each ice cream			FAT(g)	CALS
Alfresco, 1 tub			3.9	142
Billabong: Barney Banana			2.0	80
Bubbleberry			5.4	131
Chocolate Natural			2.0	80
	Chocolate Twist		6.2	141
	Triple Swirl		3.1	106
Choc'O'Malt			4.8	161
Choc. Wedge:	Choc. Malt/Spearmint/Vanilla		14.0	199
	Honeycomb		14.3	204
	Snow Wedge		13.4	204
Dixie Cup			5.5	103
Drumstick:	Mac. Nut Caramel		15.2	229
	Mint Chip		10.8	196
	Triple Choc.		12.2	214
	Vanilla		12.0	203
Eskimo Pie:	Vanilla		14.4	210
	New Eskimo Pie:	Chocolate	17.1	271
		Vanilla	18.8	284
Extra Cream Slices			5.3	95
Frosty Fruits, Tropical			<1.0	75
Frisco			11.6	199
Frozen Yoghurt:	Apricot		5.8	126
	Strawberry		5.4	129
Fruit de Light			<0.1	52
Hava Heart			15.6	223
Hazelnut Roll			12.8	187
Heaven on a Stick:	Almond		19.1	263
	Chocolate		16.7	257
	Vanilla		18.2	258
Icy Pole, all flavours average			<1.0	50
Monaco Bar			10.2	218

ICE CREAM & ICE CONFECTIONS

PAUL'S & PETER'S NOVELTY BARS - ICES		FAT(g)	CALS
Split: Pine Lime & Raspberry		2.4	76
Thumbs Up		<1.0	61
Twister:	Chocolate	8.1	172
	Strawberry, Passionfruit	7.9	174
PRITHAAGEN			
Average 125ml. serve		<0.1	90
SARA LEE 100ml. scoop			
Classic:	Berries & Cream	14.0	242
	French Vanilla	17.0	257
	Honey Pecan	19.0	234
	Honeycomb & Butterscotch	14.0	217
	Peach Mango	13.0	206
	Strawberries & Cream	13.0	214
	Ultra Chocolate	16.0	247
Classic Light:	Cappuccino Swirl	6.4	184
	French Vanilla	6.2	173
	Strawberries & Berry	6.2	171
STREETS Tubs, 100ml. scoop			
Standard:	Chocolate	4.8	89
	Strawberry	4.6	86
	Vanilla	4.7	90
Blue Ribbon:	Blueberry Cream	5.0	94
	Chocolate	5.3	92
	Toffee Cream	5.8	116
	Vanilla	5.0	92
	Light Vanilla	3.1	84
	Light Strawberry	2.8	94
Frozen Yoghurt:	Lemon	2.0	85
	Orange	1.7	89
Ice Cream Slices, 47g each		5.5	99
Sorbet:	Lemon	0.0	55
	Pine Lime	4.4	106
Super Saver: all flavours		5.1	95
Too Good To Be True:	Double Chocolate	0.5	94
	Double Toffee	0.4	93
	Vanilla & Strawberry	0.4	91
Viennetta, 100ml:	Cappuccino	8.9	137
	Chocolate	8.3	131
	Mint	8.9	122
	Vanilla	8.2	121

ICE CREAM & ICE CONFECTIONS

STREETS NOVELTY BARS - ICES each ice cream	FAT(g)	CALS
Blokka	16.7	239
Boomy	0.1	47
Bubble O'Bill	8.3	166
Calippo: Lemon	0.0	114
Orange	0.0	76
Cornetto: Choc. Mint	13.0	226
Chocolate	13.7	227
Vanilla	12.3	207
Fruit Bat	0.0	139
Fruiti Yo	1.8	90
Gaytime Golden	13.2	242
Heart: Vanilla	12.5	192
Snack Hearts (multipack), each	6.5	98
Magnum: Almond	23.1	350
Chocolate	19.4	298
Dark Classic	18.9	290
White	20.0	310
Mud Bucket Choc.	6.6	135
Oz Block, average all flavours	0.0	52
Paddle Pops: All Natural Choc. Malt	3.2	123
Banana (Nat.)	3.6	121
Chocolate	5.5	156
Rainbow	3.4	123
Siesta	3.2	101
Siesta Berry	3.2	102
Small Cup	4.7	90
Splice: Pine Lime	3.1	94
Tropical Crush	3.1	91
Sunkist	0.0	68
Super Cornetto, Fruit of the Forest	12.7	228
Super Cornetto, Toffee Crunch	13.3	238
Triple Treat	11.6	223
Vienna Chocolate	4.8	148
Yoghurt Fruit Salad	3.0	105
Yoghurt Strawberry	3.2	112
Zipp	0.0	78
SUNBURST		
Fruit Tubes, 70ml.	0.0	49
Ice Drops, all flavours, 62.5ml.	0.0	38
Sunny Boy, Razz, Glug, 150ml each	0.0	63
Zooper Doopers, 18ml. tubes	0.0	15

ICE CREAM & ICE CONFECTIONS

	FAT(g)	CALS
VITARI		
Frozen, 100ml., average all flavours	<1.0	60
Soft Serve, in Cone	<1.0	90
WEIGHT WATCHERS		
Ice Confection, 85ml. serve	1.4	57
Sweet Celebrations, 85ml. serve: Chocolate	0.3	60
Vanilla	0.2	57
WEIS		
Fruito, 80g each	2.7	109
Mango, 80g each	2.6	102
Mango mini, 40g each	1.3	51
Tropico, 80g each	6.3	134
Wildberries, 80g each	3.4	111
WENDY'S RETAIL OUTLETS		
Ice Cream, 100ml. serve, average all flavours	6.5	120
Soft Serve, 100ml.	3.3	90
Vitari Soft Serve, 100ml.	<1.0	62
Yoghurt, 100g	0.3	120
Milkshakes, 200ml. average	13.0	245
Thickshakes, 200ml. average	9.0	215
Smoothies, 200ml. average	11.0	230
Cones: plain, each	0.0	20
Waffle, each	0.5	60
WHITE WINGS		
Funny Face, each	0.0	43
Kool Pops, each	0.0	20
Space Food Sticks: Caramel	2.5	73
Chocolate	2.8	71
WOOLWORTHS - SAFEWAY		
Snow Star, 100ml. scoop	5.0	98
Velvet Cream, 100ml. scoop	5.5	103

MEALS - PIES ETC.

FROZEN MEALS	FAT(g)	CALS
N.B. Figures given are for the frozen product only. Any fat used in cooking must be added.		
ARRIBA BURRITOS		
Bean & Cheese, 200g	10.0	401
Beef & Chilli, 200g	13.6	420
Chicken & Cheese, 200g	9.8	385
Steak & Jalapeno, 200g	8.4	368
BARON'S TABLE (frozen product only)		
Chicken Kiev, each piece 175g	33.3	456
Veal Cordon Blue, each piece 138g	23.0	364
BIG BEN		
Chicken Pie, 175g	21.7	432
Country Pie, 175g	22.4	433
Extra Tasty Pie, 175g	24.9	438
Lite & Lean, 175g	20.5	399
Party Pies, 42g each	6.1	114
Steak & Onion Pie, 175g	24.2	441
Traditional Pie, 175g	24.9	438
BIRD'S EYE (frozen product only)		
Cauliflower & Cheese Bakes, 75g serve	8.9	164
Chiko Rolls, 170g each	8.7	303
Fish Cakes, 50g each	5.6	109
Vegetable Fingers, 30g each	2.3	55
For other Bird's Eye frozen products see: Fish, frozen, page 96, Vegetables/Potatoes frozen page 231		
COLONIAL FARM (frozen product only)		
Chicken Kiev, each piece, 175g	33.3	467
DEFIANCE (frozen product only)		
Cocktail pies, 38g each	5.9	108
Cocktail sausage rolls, 20g each	2.9	59
Cocktail Quiche Lorraine, 35g each	9.6	150
DOLL (frozen product only)		
Dim Sims, 13.5g each	1.0	23
Mini Spring Rolls, 18g each	1.8	43
Samosas, 15g each	3.0	49

MEALS - PIES ETC.

FROZEN MEALS	FAT(g)	CALS
FARMLAND (Frozen product only)		
Beefsteak Pie, family, ¼ whole, 125g	20.0	334
Chicken Nuggets, 20g each	3.2	64
Crunchy Fish Pie, 300g serve	18.3	343
Hamburgers, 50g each	12.1	150
Lasagne in Bechamel Sauce, ½ pack, 250g	8.3	250
Lasagne Vegetable, 300g pack	22.8	405
Macaroni Cheese, 250g	27.0	429
Meat Pie, 175g	24.2	445
Oven Fry crumbed fish fillets, each	8.9	169
Oven Fry crumbed fish fillets in lemon sauce, each	9.2	166
Party pies, 50g each	7.7	139
Sausage rolls, 42g each	7.0	102
Shepherd's pie, ¼ whole (600g), 150g	13.2	253
FINDUS		
Crispy Pancakes each pancake, 50g		
Cheese & Ham	4.0	96
Savoury Beef	8.5	156
Lean Cuisine, 1 regular pkt.:		
Beef Italienne	8.0	255
Chicken Marsala	4.0	195
Cheese Cannelloni	7.0	255
Coconut Chicken	7.0	250
Glazed Chicken	5.0	245
Macaroni Bolognese	9.0	270
Mild Vegetable Curry	8.0	250
Oriental Beef	6.0	260
Spaghetti with Beef	5.0	300
Traditional Lasagne	5.0	255
Tuna Lasagne	10.0	275
Turkey Breast	7.0	265
Zucchini Lasagne	7.0	260
Lean Cuisine Healthy Appetite, 1 pkt., 400g		
Chilli Con Carne	4.0	391
French Style Chicken	8.4	460
Indian Style Chicken Curry	11.0	456
Lean Beef Lasagne	8.4	428
Ravioli with Tomato & Olives	12.4	479
Pomes Noisettes, 100g (frozen product only)	8.2	188

MEALS - PIES ETC.

FROZEN MEALS		FAT(g)	CALS
FINDUS continued			
Red Box, 1 pkt:	Apricot Chicken Casserole, 310g	9.6	316
	Beef Teriyaki, 275g	10.0	223
	Cannelloni, 300g	18.0	360
	Lasagne Bechamel, 300g	20.0	447
	Lasagne Bolognese, 300g	14.0	378
	Macaroni & Beef, 300g	32.0	553
	Macaroni Supreme, 400g	26.0	672
	Vegetable Lasagne	11.0	351
Red Box Large Packs, each ½ packet:			
	Cannelloni, 250g	15.0	303
	Lasagne, 250g	18.0	362
	Macaroni & Cheese, 200g	18.0	346
	Potato Bake, 150g	5.3	146
	Ravioli with Tomato & Bacon, 200g	6.2	239
	Shepherd's Pie, 250g	8.0	250
Rock'n'Rolls each:			
	Beef & Vegetable	4.0	247
	Cheese & Bacon	5.0	264
	Chilli Con Carne	2.5	188
	Hawaiian Pizza	3.0	254
FOUR'N'TWENTY			
Homestyle Pies:	Chicken & Vegetable Supreme, 210g	23.1	485
	Lamb Stockpot, 210g	26.5	497
	Premium Beef, 210g	26.9	502
Light Pies:	Meat, 175g	14.0	380
	Vegetable, 175g	10.5	342
Party Pies, 50g each		7.4	133
Pasties, 175g each		21.4	412
Pies, 175g each:	Chicken	23.1	421
	Curry & Rice	23.1	442
	Meat	27.3	471
	Mexicana	22.9	442
	Pizza pie	29.9	502
	Spicy Curry	21.2	428
	Steak & Bacon	29.2	497
	Steak & Mushroom	23.3	434
	Steak & Onion	26.8	459
	Stockman's	17.9	375
	Super Meat Pie, 230g	26.7	518
	Thai Chicken & Rice	17.7	389

MEALS - PIES ETC.

FROZEN MEALS	FAT(g)	CALS
FOUR'N'TWENTY continued...		
Sausage Rolls: Bacon & Cheese, 115g	20.0	339
Regular - Jumbo, 117g each	18.5	342
Large, 80g each	12.7	238
Party size, 42g each	6.7	119
Tomato & Onion, 115g	19.0	339
Shepherd's Pie, 200g	18.6	381
GO 4 IT - MICRO EASY		
Chicken Fillet Burger	14.9	378
GRIFF'S		
Budget Gourmet, each pkt., 400g		
Beef & Black Bean	4.8	386
Beef Casserole	7.2	380
Chicken Mornay	9.2	382
Curried Prawns	4.4	293
Fried Rice, 350g	11.2	451
Homestead Beef	28.0	512
Lemon Chicken	5.6	605
Satay Prawns	13.0	455
Singapore Curry Chicken	12.0	600
Spinach & Lamb	7.2	378
Sweet & Sour Pork	22.8	665
Teriyaki Pork	7.0	467
HERBERT ADAMS		
Party Pies, 50g each	9.0	148
Pastie: plain, 175g	20.1	382
vegetable, 175g	14.0	354
Pies individual, 175g each: Heritage	22.8	438
Heritage Light	12.3	358
Meat pie	25.2	446
Meat pie Light	14.0	438
Microwave	27.3	471
Microwave Light	14.0	380
Steak & Onion	27.1	471
Pies, Family, ¼ whole, 150g serve: Meat	19.4	331
Shepherd's	13.2	272
Steak & Onion	19.5	357
Stockman's	20.3	314

FROZEN MEALS		FAT(g)	CALS
HERBERT ADAMS continued...			
Pies, Gourmet, 210g each:	Beef & Burgundy	24.2	487
	Chicken & Vegetable	25.6	506
	Lamb & Rosemary	27.1	521
Sausage Rolls, 37.5g each		6.3	108
HO - MAI (frozen product only)			
Mini Dim Sims, 3 pieces, 50g		3.3	91
Spring Rolls, 45g each		4.9	102
I & J (frozen product only)			
Bacon & Beefer Burger, 160g each		21.0	424
Beefer Burger, 150g each		21.0	396
Big Beefers, 125g each		25.1	344
Lean Beefers, 67g each		7.1	111
L'il Beefers, 50g each		10.0	138
INGHAM (frozen product only)			
Big Dippers, 10g each		1.1	35
Breast Patties, 83g each		11.4	235
Chicken Chipees, Plain/Spicy, 10g each		1.7	28
Cordon Blue, each piece, 175g		19.6	370
Fillets, 100g each		10.0	248
Kiev, each piece, 175g		28.4	425
Medallions:	Honey & Sesame, 33g each	5.0	83
	Oriental Lemon, 33g each	4.9	79
	Teriyaki, 33g each	4.5	72
Mini Drums, 67g each		9.0	203
Nuggets, 20g each		4.0	64
Parmigiana, each piece, 175g		12.4	303
Tenderloins, 100g		11.0	250
LEAN LINKS (Woolworths) (frozen product only)			
Beefburgers, 100g each		8.0	165
LOGAN FARM (frozen product only)			
Corn Nuggets, 15g each		1.3	32
LONGA-LIFE (frozen product only)			
Notburgers, 95g each		4.6	184
Notdogs, 71g each		5.3	154

MEALS - PIES ETC.

FROZEN MEALS	FAT(g)	CALS
McCAIN		
Healthy Choice Dinners, each pkt.		
Beef Medallions	5.6	226
Chicken Chasseur	3.1	251
Fillet of Lamb	6.5	251
Pepper Steak	7.8	300
Spit Roast Pork	3.1	298
Healthy Choice Entrees, each pkt.		
Apricot Chicken, 280g	4.2	299
Beef & Black Bean, 260g	3.9	291
Lamb Italian, 250g	6.3	228
Lasagne, 290g	8.7	244
Mustard Chicken, 230g	6.9	280
Satay Beef, 270g	5.7	300
Tandoori Chicken, 270g	5.1	297
Tortellini & Pumpkin Soup, 320g	9.0	237
Looney Tunes Dinners: each 200g pkt.		
Bugs Bunny Chicken Nuggets	20.6	313
Daffy Duck Spaghetti Bolognese	11.6	319
Road Runner Party Pies	21.4	436
Red Box, each pkt.		
Agnolotti Napoli, 350g	15.8	441
Beef Hotpot, 400g	10.4	344
Curried Prawns, 350g	2.0	315
Fettuccine Carbonara, 375g	31.5	574
Fried Rice, 350g	7.7	392
Lasagne, 400g	27.0	620
Lasagne Large (750g pkt.), ½ pkt., 375g	25.4	582
Roast Beef, 320g	5.4	282
Roast Chicken, 320g	7.7	351
Roast Lamb, 320g	6.0	289
Roast Pork, 320g	5.1	326
Roast Turkey, 320g	11.5	314
Shepherd's Pie, 400g	22.4	464
Spaghetti Bolognese, 400g	13.2	472
Steak Diane, 320g	8.3	266
Sweet & Sour Chicken, 350g	10.9	438
Veal Cordon Bleu, 320g	28.8	518
Vegetable Croquettes, 100g	13.3	210

MEALS - PIES ETC.

FROZEN MEALS		FAT(g)	CALS
McMAIN			
Tastee:	Traditional Meat Pie, 170g each	21.3	445
	175g, (4 per pkt)	21.9	458
	Meat & Mushy Pie, 190g	19.4	543
	Chicken Sausage Roll, 100g	16.0	271
	Monster Sausage Roll, 120g	19.8	332
MUNCH'N'CRUNCH			
	Beef & Vegetable Pie, 150g	17.6	354
	Chicken & Vegetable Pie, 150g	17.7	361
NANNA'S			
	Asparagus Rolls, 29g each	4.5	75
	Sausage Rolls, 29g each	4.1	77
NATIONAL			
	Individual Meat Pie	32.0	267
NICHIREI (frozen product only)			
	Prawn Cutlets, 25g each	0.6	44
	Tempura Prawns, 100g	12.5	210
PAMPAS			
	Beefsteak Pie, ¼ whole, 150g (600g Family)	13.7	283
	Chicken & Veg Pie, ¼ whole, 125g (500g Family)	13.9	283
	Shepherd's Pie, ¼ whole, 175g (700g Family)	8.2	240
PAPA GUISEPPE			
	Quiche Lorraine, ¼ whole, 125g	25.0	413
	Quiche Light, ¼ whole, 125g	16.0	288
	Spinach & Cheese Quiche Singles, 125g each	16.0	288
	Pizzas..*see Page 172*		
SARA LEE			
Quiches:	Quiche Lorraine, ¼ whole, 150g serve	33.0	438
	Quiche Lorraine Mini, 120g each	24.0	354
	Vegetable, ¼ whole, 150g serve	27.0	391
	Tasmanian Salmon Fans, 33.3g each	2.8	54
	Viennese Fans, 33.3g each	2.7	58
	Viennese-Rosti, 33.3g each: Cheese	3.0	66
	Plain	3.2	63
	Pumpkin	3.7	63

MEALS - PIES ETC.

FROZEN MEALS	FAT(g)	CALS
SARGENT'S & SCOTT'S		
Chicken & Vegetable Pie, 175g each	19.8	405
Meat Pie/Curried Meat Pie, 175g each	19.5	382
Meat & Vegetable Pie, 175g each	20.5	385
Party Pies, 54g each, average	6.0	118
Steak & Mushroom Pie, 175g each	20.1	401
Steak & Onion, 175g each	20.6	405
STEGGLES (frozen product only)		
Chicken Burger, 85g each	13.0	309
Chicken Nuggets, 20g each	3.3	54
Chicken Rissoles, 85g each	11.1	173
Chicken Rissoles, Mini, 40g each	5.2	81
Chicken Sausages, 85g each	8.6	140
Crumbed Breast Fillets, 120g each	8.3	215
Crumbed Drumsticks, 145g each	16.7	314
Crunchy Chicken Fries, 70g each	13.0	193
Honey Wing Sticks, 50g each	8.5	117
Potato Crumbed Nuggets, 20g each	3.0	51
Pre-Cooked Frozen Products:		
Burgers, 83g each	11.7	209
Crumbed Potato Nuggets, 20g each	3.5	58
Nuggets (chicken), 20g each	3.4	91
Royales, 100g	17.1	276
Krisp Bakes, 100g	5.5	185
WEDGEWOOD		
Beef Croquettes, 50g each	4.3	106
Party Pasties, 42g each	6.6	113
Party Pies, 50g each	7.7	137
Pasties, 170g each	20.7	400
Pies, 170g each: Chicken	22.4	429
Curry & Rice	22.4	409
Meat	26.5	458
Mexicana	22.3	429
Steak & Mushroom	22.6	421
Sausage Rolls: Partysize, 42g each	6.7	119
Large, 80g each	12.2	229
Jumbo, 115g each	18.0	348
Savoury Nibbles, 11.5g each	1.9	29
Vol-au-Vents, 17g each: Chicken	3.5	52
Egg & Bacon/Mexicana	4.5	58
Hawaiian	4.1	54

MEALS - PIES ETC.

PACKET & CANNED

N.B. Some values are given for dry product only (you will need to add the values for any added meat etc.) plus some values are for product made as directed.

TIP *Where values are given for products 'made as directed' eg: Pasta & Sauce mixes, you can decrease the fat and calorie contents by substituting skim milk for whole milk and deleting any fat (margarine/butter) that the packet says to add.*

CONTINENTAL	FAT(g)	CALS
Asian Noodles ¼ pkt., dry (not made up):		
Chow Mein	1.1	104
Honey Soy	0.8	125
Indonesian Satay	2.4	131
Singapore Curry	1.6	112
Spicy Plum	1.1	127
Sweet & Sour	1.1	129
Thai Curry	1.5	112
Creamy Potato Strips 130g serve, made as directed:		
with Bacon	5.5	150
with Sour Cream & Chives	6.2	160
with Tasty Cheese	5.9	150
Easy Meals 1 pkt., dry mix only (add values for any meat etc. added):		
Apricot Chicken Curry	1.5	180
Beef Strogonoff	5.5	175
Chicken Chasseur	1.9	128
Chicken Supreme Pie, 127g pack	28.7	591
Chilli Con Carne	1.6	141
Chow Mein	2.4	104
Cottage Pie	9.0	504
Creamy Tuna Mornay	7.4	241
Harvest Beef Pie, 202g pack	19.8	853
Indian Chicken Rice	7.9	157
Indonesian Beef Stirfry	9.5	177
Lamb Ragout	0.9	163
Malaysian Creamy Satay	4.1	143
Mild Mince Curry	6.4	187
Mild Thai Curry	7.9	191
Oriental Beef with Cashews	4.3	194
Rich Beefy Mince	1.6	188
Savoury Tuna & Tomato	1.0	208
Sicilian Mince	1.3	139
Spaghetti Bolognese	1.2	200

MEALS - PIES ETC.

PACKET & CANNED	FAT(g)	CALS
CONTINENTAL		
Easy Meals continued...		
Tangy Sweet & Sour	0.6	227
Tomato & Herb Sausages	1.9	141
Tuna & Broccoli Bake	1.5	125
Pasta & Sauce, ½ cup, made as directed:		
Alfredo, 124g	9.0	190
Chicken Curry, 124g	8.2	170
Creamy Bacon Carbonara, 123g	8.1	180
Creamy Marinara, 128g	6.8	170
Creamy Pomodoro, 140g	3.1	140
Creamy Vegetable Fontana, 140g	3.6	140
Fettuccini Verdi, 120g	8.6	190
Korma Vegetable Curry, 140g	2.6	130
Macaroni Cheese, 120g	7.0	180
Mushroom & Wine, 110g	6.2	160
Penne Florentine, 120g	7.2	180
Romano Tricolore, 100g ⅓ cup	6.9	150
Savoury Tomato & Onion, 120g ½ cup	6.5	170
Sour Cream & Chives, 118g	7.8	170
Sour Cream & Mushroom, 115g	7.0	170
Sour Cream & Pumpkin, 140g	3.8	150
Potato Hash Brown's, 70g serve, (2 hash browns):		
All flavours	10.0	180
Potato Patties 100g serve, made as directed:		
Bubble & Squeak	5.6	140
with Bacon & Cheese/Sour Cream & Chives	5.7	140
with Cheese & Onion	5.6	150
with Spring Vegetables	5.6	140
Rices: ¼ pkt, made as directed:		
Cheesy Risotto, ½ cup 95g	6.0	170
Chicken & Sweetcorn, ½ cup 95g	4.4	150
Chicken & Vegetable, ½ cup 90g	5.0	155
Garden Herb, ½ cup 95g	4.5	150
Oriental Fried Rice, ½ cup 105g	6.6	210
Rices of The World: ¼ pkt., made as directed (rice only):		
Chinese	1.2	121
Creole	1.8	133
Hawaiian	2.1	137
Indian	1.9	130
Satay	2.8	142
Thai	1.0	120

MEALS - PIES ETC.

PACKET & CANNED	FAT(g)	CALS
EDGELL		
Quick & Healthy, 212g ctn:		
Thai Stir Fry	3.4	155
Quick & Hot, 212g ctn:		
Baked Beans & Franks	4.7	193
Cheesy Macaroni	15.7	290
Spaghetti Bolognese	6.1	191
Quick Shots, 212g ctn:		
Asparagus & Turkey	13.1	212
Beef Raviolini	5.3	191
Chicken Tortellini	9.5	212
Farmhouse Hot Pot	5.7	210
Pasta & Beef Strogonoff	11.0	244
Penne Bolognese	8.3	189
Quick Shots, 310g ctn:		
Beef Raviolini	7.8	279
Chicken Tortellini	14.0	310
Farmhouse Hot Pot	8.4	307
FARMLAND		
Pasta & Sauce 100g serve, made as directed:		
Alfredo	9.2	162
Carbonara	9.3	182
Creamy Curry	8.0	161
Sour Cream & Chives	9.1	180
Macaroni Cheese	9.7	190
GREEN'S		
Meals in Minutes, made up as directed:		
Beef Penang, 150g serve	1.7	186
Rice & Vegetables, 150g serve	1.2	181
Singapore Noodles, 110g serve	0.9	110
Potato Mixes made up as directed, 100g serve:		
Bacon & Herb	12.6	167
Cheddar Cheese	5.0	120
Sour Cream & Chives	5.0	122
HARVEST, ½ can, 212.5g (425g can):		
Beef Ravioli with Tomato Sauce	3.6	164
Curried Vegetables & Sausages	6.8	171
Irish Stew	4.7	132
Mild Curry	3.6	143

MEALS - PIES ETC.

PACKET & CANNED	FAT(g)	CALS
HARVEST continued...		
Mushrooms & Steak	2.6	118
Onions & Braised Steak	1.7	127
Onions, Steak & Kidney	2.3	139
Sweet & Sour Pork	3.9	151
Vegetables & Sausages	3.2	131
Vegetables & Steak	1.7	118
HEINZ		
Baked Beans, ½ can, 220g (440g can):		
in Tomato Sauce/Salt Reduced	1.5	203
in Bar-B-Q Sauce	5.5	247
in Ham Sauce	4.4	245
Baked Beans Plus, ½ can, 220g (440g can):		
Boston Style	1.1	242
Italian Style	2.4	225
Mexican Style	2.8	235
Spanish Style	0.9	216
Kids Cuisine, whole can, 225g:		
Farmhouse Chicken Casserole	5.2	183
Macaroni Steak Dinner	6.0	178
Pasta & Chicken Supreme	8.1	219
Savoury Rice with Beef	1.6	183
Spaghetti Bolognese	3.6	151
Spaghetti, ½ can, 220g (440g can):		
Alphaghetti, per 225g can	1.8	149
Bolognese	1.1	117
in Tomato Sauce & Cheese/salt reduced	1.3	135
Spaghetti Oops, 130g can	1.3	86
Spooky Spaghetti, 220g	1.8	145
Wholemeal Spaghetti, 220g	1.5	143
Supersnacks, whole can, 225g:		
Chunky Vegetable & Beef	2.5	147
Ravioli Bolognese	6.3	221
Rice & Beef Curry	9.9	259
Spaghetti Bolognese	4.8	167
Tortellini Bolognese	4.0	176
Vegetable Beef Casserole	8.1	228
Vegetable Chicken Casserole	6.0	167
Vegetable Lamb Hot Pot	8.6	221
Vegetables, Steak & Kidney	13.0	255

MEALS - PIES ETC.

PACKET & CANNED	FAT(g)	CALS
HOLBROOKS		
Dinner Winner, ¼ pkt., dry (ADD values for any added meat etc.):		
Beef	0.8	165
Curry	1.1	177
Savoury Tomato	0.8	165
Rice-A-Riso: average all flavours, 1 pkt.	1.0	230
HOME GOURMET		
Rice Dinners, 67g serve, made as directed:		
Chinese Claypot Beef	2.9	200
Sambal Prawn Coconut	8.2	238
Spicy Chicken	8.3	245
KARMA GOURMET CUISINE		
Authentic Indian Chicken Korma, 300g	25.2	277
Authentic Indian Lamb Madras, 300g	21.6	375
Traditional Indian Beef Curry	17.4	333
KRAFT		
Tinned Meals, ½ can, 220g (440g can):		
Irish Stew	7.0	181
Ravioli	11.4	257
Spaghetti & Meatballs	9.9	218
Spaghetti Bolognese	11.7	226
Vegetables & Sausages, 210g	12.2	207
Packet Pasta Meals, made as directed:		
Cheese & Bacon, 180g serve	12.8	276
Cheese & Tomato, 170g serve	11.6	241
Macaroni & Cheese, 230g serve	14.5	352
Macaroni & Cheese Deluxe, 270g serve	32.4	583
Snack, Braised Steak & Onions, 220g serve	14.7	289
LONGA LIFE, Vegetarian Products		
Cavellami, 30g	0.3	35
Kaiser Royale, 30g	3.2	68
NotBacon, 1 rasher, 14.6g	2.1	39
Notburgers (frozen), 95g each	4.6	184
Notdogs (frozen), 71g each	5.3	154
NotPepperoni, 1 stick, 25g	3.8	38
Vege Chicken, 30g	2.9	69
Vege Garlic, 30g	2.6	84

MEALS - PIES ETC.

PACKET & CANNED	FAT(g)	CALS
LONGA LIFE, Vegetarian Products continued...		
Vege Ham, 30g	4.1	64
Vege Henchen, 30g	1.8	99
Vege Herb, 30g	1.5	64
Vege Hotdogs, 63g each	2.3	102
Vege Kabana, 30g	1.9	67
Vege Party Franks, 31g each	1.1	50
Vege Smoke, 30g	2.5	89
Vege Sausages, 63g each	2.5	103
Vege Sausages, curried, 63g each	2.3	105
Vege Schnitzel, 30g	0.6	63
Vege Wurst, 30g	2.6	66
MAGGI		
2 minute noodles, made as directed:		
average all flavours, 1 pkt	15.0	385
Rice'n'More, made as directed:		
average all flavours, 100g	4.0	364
Potatoes'n'More, 100g, made as directed:		
Cheese & Bacon	3.9	343
Creamy Cheese	4.0	364
Double Cheese	3.7	354
McCORMICK		
Dinner Mixes 1 pkt., dry:		
Country Chicken	1.1	111
Italian	1.3	135
Mexican	0.8	189
Satay	2.6	136
Sweet & Sour	0.4	147
Tuna/Salmon pattie mix, 1 pkt., dry	3.0	139
NO FRILLS		
Pasta & Sauce, 100g, made as directed:		
Alfredo	7.9	164
Bacon Carbonara	9.7	163
Sour Cream & Chives	5.4	157
NUTAL		
Vegetarian Burgers, average all flavours, 1, 12g each	9.9	262

MEALS - PIES ETC.

PACKET & CANNED	FAT(g)	CALS
OLD EL PASO		
Corn Chips, 100g	34.0	556
Dips: Chunky Tomato Salsa, 1 Tbsp., 20g	<0.1	8
Bean & Tomato Salsa, 1 Tbsp., 20g	<0.1	17
Mexe Beans, 100g	0.4	84
Nachos Topping, 100g	<0.1	67
Refried Beans, all flavours, 100g	0.8	81
Seasoning Mixes: Burrito, 100g (in dinner packs)	2.6	322
Chilli, 35g	1.6	100
Taco, 35g	1.0	93
Taco Shells: Regular, 11g each	2.9	54
Super, 18g each	4.3	86
Taco Sauce, all flavours, 100g	<0.1	31
Thick & Chunky Salsa, all flavours, 100g	<0.1	27
Tostaco Trays, 22g each	6.3	111
PATAKS		
Tinned Meals, 200g (½ 400g can):		
Khabli Chana Dhal	9.4	226
Lobhia Dhal	7.4	204
Moong Dhal	7.6	228
Vegetable Curry Aloo Mattar Sabzi	2.4	172
Vegetable Curry Sabzi Tarkari	1.8	152
PLUMROSE, *(also see Meat/Smallgoods page 158)*		
Canned Frankfurts, 50g each	8.0	100
Cocktail frankfurts, 16g each	2.6	32
Hot Dogs, 79g each	12.6	158
P.M.U.		
Tinned Meals, 225g can:		
Baked Beans in Tomato Sauce	0.9	214
Curried Rice & Steak	5.2	201
Rice Steak & Onions	9.7	187
Spaghetti in Tomato Sauce & Cheese	1.6	122
Vegetables & Steak	7.9	196
Tinned Meals, 130g can:		
Curried Baked Beans	1.3	129
Curried Spaghetti	1.1	76
RICE-A-RISO		
¼ pkt., dry, average all flavours	1.0	230

MEALS - PIES ETC.

PACKET & CANNED	FAT(g)	CALS
SANITARIUM		
Vegetarian Products:		
BBQ Links, 42.5g each	5.0	70
Bologna, 1 slice, 30g	2.8	62
Casserole Mince, ½ can, 215g (430g can)	1.3	172
Country Stew, ½ can, 215g (430g can)	6.9	161
Lima Beans, ½ can, 215g (430g can)	0.9	172
Nutmeat, 1 slice, 54g (1/8 430g can)	4.4	103
Nutolene, 1 slice, 54g (1/8 430g can)	10.0	124
Rediburger, ¼ can, 108g (430g can)	4.2	178
Salad Loaf, 100g	6.2	125
Savoury Brown Lentils, ½ can, 215g (430g can)	0.7	129
Savoury Pie, 110g serve (¼ can)	9.7	198
Soy Beans Natural, ½ can, 215g (430g can)	6.2	151
Soy Beans in Tomato Sauce, ½ can, 215g (430g can)	6.9	194
Soya Loaf, 100g	9.8	185
Swiss Rounds, pattie, 110g each	7.0	165
Tender Bits, ½ can, 215g (430g can)	1.9	183
Vege Cuts, 2 slices, 72g	1.2	76
Vegelinks, 37.5g each	2.2	51
Vegetarian Nugget Mix, made as directed, 100g	5.5	160
Vegetarian Sausage Roll Mix, made as directed, 100g	2.9	125
Vegetarian Sausages, 42.5g each	1.9	53
Gravy Quik, 1 Tbsp., 10g	0.6	33
TVP Chunks, dry, 1 Tbsp., 22g (makes ½ cup)	0.6	66
TVP Mince, dry, 1 Tbsp,. 22g (makes ½ cup)	0.5	66
Vita Burger, dry, 1 Tbsp., 22g (makes ½ cup)	0.5	66
SAN REMO		
La Pasta, made as directed, ¼ pkt., 125g:		
Spicy Tomato & Herbs	5.2	136
All other flavours, average	6.6	158
SOY FEAST, Vegetarian Products		
Burger Mix, ¼ pkt., 50g (approx. 2 patties)	1.3	168
Taco Mix, ¼ pkt., 50g (fills approx. 3 tacos)	0.9	162
S.P.C.		
Baked Beans, ½ can, 220g (440g can)	1.8	207
Spaghetti, ½ can, 220g (440g can)	2.4	146

MEALS - PIES ETC.

PACKET & CANNED	FAT(g)	CALS
SUIMIN		
Each Cup, average all flavours	17.0	360
TOM PIPER, ½ can, 200g (400g can):		
Braised Steak & Onions	5.0	203
Bolognese Mince with Pasta	10.4	196
Chicken & Pasta Supreme	8.6	182
Chicken Hot Pot	5.6	139
Creamy Tomato, Chicken & Pasta	4.8	177
Curried Mince with Vegetables	11.2	205
Farmhouse Mince	18.0	268
Hawaiian Chicken	3.0	173
Irish Stew	8.0	162
Lamb Casserole	7.6	189
Sausages, Tomato & Onion	11.8	211
Savoury Mince & Vegetables	12.4	201
Sweet Curry	7.2	182
Vegetables & Braised Steak	5.0	156
Vegetables & Sausages	8.8	186
1 whole small can, 210g:		
Braised Steak & Onions	5.3	214
Vegetables & Braised Steak	5.3	164
UNCLE BEN'S		
Made as directed, 100g serve:		
Rice with: Broccoli & Cheese	3.2	140
Chicken & Vegetable	2.2	117
Green Beans & Almonds	3.6	181
Long Grain & Wild Rice with Mushrooms	2.3	185
VEGE BURGER		
Made as directed, with egg, 100g	6.0	190
Made as directed, without egg (plus oil), 100g	14.0	275
VESTA, ½ packet serve, made as directed:		
Beef Curry	7.0	427
Chicken Curry	7.6	422
Chicken Supreme	12.7	477
Nasi Goreng	4.2	386
Paella	2.7	358
Prawn Curry	5.1	374

MEALS - PIES ETC.

PACKET & CANNED	FAT(g)	CALS
VETTA		
Noodles Plus, 100g serve, made as directed:		
Chinese Chicken	3.9	135
Chow Mein	3.9	135
Indonesian Goreng	4.1	140
Satay	6.7	169
Pasta Plus, ½ cup, made as directed:		
Alfredo, 145g	7.8	260
Carbonara, 145g	7.3	190
Chicken Curry, 140g	6.9	185
Chicken & Mushroom, 145g	6.8	185
Creamy Vegetable, 120g	7.5	200
Rice Plus, 100g serve, made as directed:		
Chinese Chicken	5.1	175
Fried Rice	6.3	205
Pilaf	5.7	180
WATTIES		
Baked Beans, 100g serve:		
Plain	0.4	117
and Bacon	3.8	147
and Meatballs	2.5	130
and Sausages	3.3	141
Chilli Beans	0.2	48
Quick & Tasty, ½ can, 220g (440g can):		
Chilli Con Carne	4.7	262
Pasta Spirals	3.9	179
Spaghetti Bolognese	7.0	264
Steak & Onion	10.9	246
Steak & Vegetables	10.9	260
Tomato Ravioli	4.6	233
Spaghetti, 100g serve:		
Plain	0.3	72
and Bacon	4.0	109
Italian Style	0.3	70
and Meatballs	2.4	87
and Sausages	3.2	97

MEALS - PIES ETC.

PACKET & CANNED	FAT(g)	CALS
WEIGHT WATCHERS		
Pasta Portions, 100g, made as directed:		
Creamy Mushroom	1.8	113
Macaroni Cheese	2.1	113
Mild Creamy Curry	1.9	115
Napolitana	1.3	110
WHITE WINGS		
Noodles of the East, ¼ pkt., made as directed:		
Chinese Chicken/Chow Mein	4.1	140
Honey Lemon	4.4	160
Indonesian Goreng	4.1	140
Teriyaki	4.1	145
Thai Curry	4.3	145
Pasta Plus, ½ cup serve, made as directed:		
Alfredo	7.8	260
Cheese & Herb	6.8	185
Cheese & Tomato	7.0	190
Chicken Curry	6.9	185
Chicken & Mushroom	6.8	185
Creamy Mushroom	6.8	190
Carbonara	7.3	190
Tomato & Herb	2.9	150
Quick Fried Rice, average all flavours, 60g	4.0	125
WOOLWORTHS		
Pasta Mixes, 100g serve, made as directed:		
Alfredo	7.9	164
Bacon Carbonara	9.7	167
Macaroni Cheese	10.7	207
Sour Cream & Chives	5.4	157

MEAT

The fat values for meat and thus the calorie values also, vary greatly depending on whether the purchased piece of meat is trimmed of all it's fat or not. Therefore, figures are given for meat that is consumed with all of it's fat and also for meat that is trimmed of all of it's fat. You will notice a large difference!

(A great way to instantly cut the amount of fat in your diet is to only eat meat that has been trimmed of all it's visible fat either by your butcher or yourself!)

Note: Meat loses moisture and fat when it is cooked and therefore it also loses weight (this can vary from 20-50%). So, when you bring your meat home from the butcher it is a good idea to weigh each serving either before or after you cook it. (You may have bought a 150g steak home from the shop - but after you have grilled it, the steak will weigh considerably less - perhaps 115-120 grams).

Where figures are given for raw meat the weight specified eg. 100g is the weight of the meat as purchased.

Where figures are given for cooked meat (eg. grilled) the weight specified eg. 100g is the weight of the meat AFTER cooking (ie. you would have purchased a piece of meat around 130g to end up with a cooked product weighing 100g).

BEEF		**FAT(g)**	**CALS**
Average all cuts, Grilled:			
Small Steak (100g raw)	Fatty as purchased	9.5	166
	Lean only	4.4	127
Medium Steak (150g raw)	Fatty as purchased	15.0	265
	Lean only	7.0	204
Large Steak (200g raw)	Fatty as purchased	20.3	356
	Lean only	9.5	273

Various Cuts: (Each cut is shown firstly as 100g raw weight so that a comparison can be made between various cuts. Each cut is also shown as a cooked weight approximating the average serving size for that particular cut, eg. Fillet steak is usually smaller than Rump.)

Beef Offal: *see Offal page 157*

			FAT(g)	CALS
Blade:	100g raw	- Fatty	10.8	179
		- Lean Only	5.0	129
	100g grilled	- Fatty	10.6	206
		- Lean Only	6.8	176

MEAT

BEEF Various Cuts			FAT(g)	CALS
Brisket: (corned beef) raw 100g		- Fatty	14.7	200
		- Lean Only	1.6	94
	100g boiled	- Fatty	23.4	313
		- Lean Only	9.7	212
Chuck Steak:	100g raw	- Fatty	8.7	156
		- Lean Only	2.9	108
	190g cooked (1 cup diced):			
		- Fatty	26.0	487
		- Lean Only	11.4	284
Fillet Steak:	100g raw	- Fatty	10.7	177
		- Lean Only	4.2	124
	70g grilled	- Fatty	9.2	163
		- Lean Only	5.8	137
Rib Steak:	100g raw	- Fatty	21.1	263
		- Lean Only	3.8	121
	112g grilled (raw weight 150g):			
		- Fatty	24.6	339
		- Lean Only	6.3	197
Ribeye Steak:	100g raw	- Fatty	11.9	191
		- Lean Only	4.4	132
	130g grilled (175g raw):			
		- Fatty	20.7	334
		- Lean Only	10.4	256
Round Steak:	100g raw	- Fatty	9.1	162
		- Lean Only	3.7	117
	150g grilled (200g raw):			
		- Fatty	14.4	305
		- Lean Only	9.3	264
Rump Steak:	100g raw	- Fatty	16.7	230
		- Lean Only	2.6	117
	150g grilled (medium)	- Fatty	25.2	405
		- Lean Only	10.0	287
	200g grilled (large)	- Fatty	33.6	540
		- Lean Only	13.4	382
Silverside:	100g raw	- Fatty	11.7	187
		- Lean Only	2.2	109
	100g baked - 2 slices	- Fatty	11.7	231
		- Lean Only	4.6	177

MEAT

BEEF Various Cuts			FAT(g)	CALS
Corned:	100g raw	- Fatty	7.3	130
		- Lean Only	1.1	79
	100g boiled - 2 slices	- Fatty	12.9	204
		- Lean Only	3.5	129
Sirloin:	100g raw	- Fatty	17.2	232
		- Lean Only	5.9	138
	130g grilled (175g raw):			
		- Fatty	25.0	358
		- Lean Only	11.4	250
Skirt:	100g raw	- Fatty	3.7	122
		- Lean Only	2.4	112
	100g boiled	- Fatty	6.2	196
		- Lean Only	4.9	187
Topside Roast:	100g raw	- Fatty	6.7	144
		- Lean Only	3.2	115
	100g baked - 2 slices	- Fatty	10.0	191
		- Lean Only	4.9	151

BEEF MINCE

To keep fat to a minimum always try to choose the leanest mince.

TIP: *Purchase a lean cut of steak and have your butcher trim it of all fat and then mince it for you.*

	FAT(g)	CALS
Fatty: (15 - 17% fat)		
eg. hamburger mince, 100g raw	16.1	222
Lean: (6 - 7% fat)		
eg. Topside Mince, 100g raw	6.7	144
Medium Fat: (10 - 11% fat)		
100g raw	11.0	178
Hamburger Patties:		
Homemade:		
Calculate by weighing the amount of mince used in each pattie:		
eg. using 75g lean mince...	5.0	108
(plus fat used in cooking!!)		

Frozen: see Frozen Meals, page 130.

MEAT

LAMB	**FAT(g)**	**CALS**

As for beef, many cuts of lamb contain a lot of excess fat. Try to trim all visible fat from lamb cuts. New Trim Lamb cuts are all pre-trimmed and are low in fat.

Various Cuts

	FAT(g)	CALS
Breast Roll, baked, stuffed, 100g - 2 slices	21.5	291
Chump Chops: 1 chop raw, approx 100g incl. bones		
- Fatty	28.0	305
- Lean Only	5.0	120
1 chop grilled, 85g incl. bones (approx.)		
- Fatty	12.0	185
- Lean only	4.4	115
Cutlets (Ribloin chops):		
1 cutlet, raw, 50g incl. bones - Fatty	13.9	150
- Lean Only	1.7	39
1 cutlet, grilled/baked, 40g incl. bones		
- Fatty	10.0	130
- Lean Only	2.5	58
Lamb Offal: *see Offal Page 157*		
Leg: Baked/Roast, 2 slices - 100g - Fatty	11.9	224
- Lean Only	5.6	176
Mid-Loin Chops:		
1 chop raw, approx. 85g incl. bones - Fatty	22.2	244
- Lean Only	1.8	60
1 chop, grilled, 65g incl. bones - Fatty	15.1	180
- Lean Only	2.5	65
Neck Chops: raw, no bone, 100g - Fatty	27.0	310
- Lean Only	5.3	130
stewed/simmered, ½ cup, 100g		
- Fatty	27.5	356
- Lean Only	13.7	253
Shank: raw, average size incl. bones, 250g		
- Fatty	10.8	191
- Lean Only	2.0	121
stewed/simmered, meat only, 100g		
- Fatty	10.5	223
- Lean Only	4.5	179
Shoulder: Baked/Roast, 2 slices - 100g		
- Fatty	20.7	290
- Lean Only	7.1	186

MEAT

TRIM LAMB		FAT(g)	CALS

Figures given are for a 100g serving of COOKED trim lamb, edible portions only, lean meat only.

		FAT(g)	CALS
Butterfly Steak: grilled		9.6	203
Round Steak: grilled		8.5	187
Topside Steak: grilled		7.2	189
Lamb Fillet: grilled		6.8	170
Diced/Strips: stir fried		7.5	179
Roasts:	Round, dry roasted/microwaved	6.1	160
	Eye of Loin, dry roasted/microwaved	6.6	166
	Topside, dry roasted/microwaved	5.9	158
	Silvertop, dry roasted/microwaved	5.0	151
Schnitzel:	Round, pan fried	6.3	165
	Topside, pan fried	5.6	160
Mince:	dry fried (using no fat)	8.5	174

PORK

Only cooked weights are given (25-30% less than purchased raw weight of meat).

Various Cuts

		FAT(g)	CALS
Forequarter Chops: 1 chop, grilled, average 150g (200g raw)			
	- Fatty	32.5	395
	- Lean Only	12.5	210
Leg: Roast/Baked, 2 slices - 100g	- Fatty	26.7	341
	- Lean Only	4.0	170
Mid-Loin Chops: 1 chop grilled, average 150g			
	- Fatty	33.5	400
	- 75% Lean	11.4	200
Spareribs: roast, edible portion, 50g (approx. 3 ribs)			
	- Fatty	19.0	220
	- 75% Lean	5.5	160

New Fashioned Pork Cuts

These cuts are generally much lower in fat than the regular cuts.

		FAT(g)	CALS
Butterfly Steak: grilled 100g	- Fatty	17.6	262
	- Lean Only	4.7	161
Leg Steak: grilled 100g	- Fatty	5.9	172
	- Lean Only	3.5	147
Medallion Steak: grilled 100g	- Fatty	22.6	311
	- Lean Only	6.3	186
Other Pork Cuts:	Pork Crackling, 30g	8.5	145
	Pigs Trotters, 1	15.5	165

MEAT

PORK			FAT(g)	CALS
Pork Offal, *see Offal, page 157*				
Pork Pie, average	- Small (8 cm. diameter), 175g		46.0	650
	- Large (12cm. diameter), 435g		110.0	1600
Pork Mince, from a new fashioned pork cut:				
	- 100g (approx. 18% fat)		17.5	260

BACON & HAM

			FAT(g)	CALS
Middle Rashers, 1 rasher, average, 35g:				
	Grilled	- Fat left on	6.7	100
		- Lean Only	3.7	70
	Fried	- Fat left on	10.3	130
		- Lean Only	4.8	75
Ham Steaks: average 110g each, grilled			8.6	179
Bacon Bits: 1 tspn., 5g			0.9	15
Ham - *see Cold Meats, page 158*				

VEAL

			FAT(g)	CALS
Average all cuts:	100g raw	- Fatty	3.5	120
		- Lean Only	1.5	103
	100g cooked	- Fatty	3.9	158
		- Lean Only	2.5	148
Forequarter:	100g raw	- Fatty	5.4	136
		- Lean Only	2.0	107
	100g cooked (approx. ½ cup)			
		- Fatty	5.2	186
		- Lean Only	3.2	172
Leg:	100g raw	- Fatty	1.5	98
		- Lean Only	0.3	87
Roast/Baked	100g - 2 slices	- Fatty	1.6	141
		- Lean Only	0.9	135
Leg Steak:	100g raw	- Fatty	2.7	116
		- Lean Only	1.8	109
average steak, fried, 65g		- Fatty	2.5	103
		- Lean Only	2.0	100
Loin Chops:	100g raw	- Fatty	4.5	130
		- Lean Only	1.5	104
1 chop, grilled approx. 110g raw weight incl. bones				
		- Fatty	2.7	87
		- Lean Only	1.5	79

MEAT

VEAL

			FAT(g)	CALS
Shank:	100g raw, meat only	- Fatty	2.4	106
		- Lean Only	0.4	89
	100g stewed, ½ cup	- Fatty	6.6	178
		- Lean Only	2.4	145
Schnitzel:	Crumbed, grilled, average serve 150g			
		- Fatty	6.5	235
		- Lean Only	4.8	215
	Crumbed, fried, 150g serve			
		- Fatty	22.0	370
		- Lean Only	20.0	350
Shoulder Steak:	100g raw	- Fatty	4.3	129
		- Lean Only	2.5	113
	75g grilled, average serve			
		- Fatty	3.2	115
		- Lean Only	2.4	108

Veal Offal: *see Offal page 157*

SAUSAGES

			FAT(g)	CALS
Beef:	Thin, 45g each	grilled	8.2	116
		fried	8.8	128
	Thick, 75g each	grilled	12.7	181
		fried	13.1	200
Pork:	Thin, 45g each	grilled	9.8	129
		fried	10.6	140
	Thick, 75g each	grilled	15.2	201
		fried	16.0	220
Lean Links:	Sausages, 60g each		<6.0	96
	Bar-B-Q Sausages, 63g each		6.0	101
Frankfurts,	average, 75g each, boiled		15.0	190
	cocktail size, 30g each, boiled		4.5	57
	Canned (**Plumrose**):			
	Frankfurts, 50g each		8.0	100
	Cocktail Frankfurts, 16g each		2.6	32
	Hot Dogs, 79g each		12.6	158
	Four & Twenty, Hot Dogs, 150g each		21.3	396
	Lean Links, low fat frankfurts, 63g each		6.0	101
Longa Life:	Vege sausages, 63g, each average all flavours		2.4	104
	Vegetarian Notdogs, 70g each		5.2	152
	Vegetarian Party Franks, 31g each		1.1	50
Nutri-Lean:	100g		3.0	108

MEAT

SAUSAGES	FAT(g)	CALS
Sanitarium Vegetarian Sausages:		
Bar-B-Q Links, 42.5g each	5.0	70
Sausages, 42.5g each	1.9	53
Vegelinks, 38g each,	2.2	51
Saveloy: battered, deep fried, 1	21.0	310

RABBIT

100g raw, incl.bone	5.2	120
100g baked, incl. bone	6.5	163
100g stewed, no bone	7.7	188

GAME, GOURMET & SPECIALTY

Buffalo: 100g cooked	1.0	150
Caviar: Red 1 Tbsp., 19g	1.6	30
Black 1 Tbsp., 19g	1.0	18
Crocodile: 100g cooked	1.0	175
Frogs Legs: fried, 2 medium	2.5	185
Grouse: 100g roasted (incl. bone)	4.4	115
Kangaroo: 100g cooked, lean rump	1.5	105
Pheasant: 100g roasted (incl. bone), no skin	6.0	134
Pigeon: 100g roasted (incl. bone)	5.6	100
100g breast, roasted (no bone)	13.0	230
Quail/Spatchcock: 100g roasted (incl. bone)	7.0	170
Snails (Escargots):		
raw, 15g each	0.0	15
in garlic butter, ½ dozen	16.0	230
Turtle: raw, 100g	0.5	110
turtle egg, 100g	12.0	212
Venison: 100g roast,	6.5	200
100g roast, extra lean	4.8	150
Witchetty Grubs: 1 medium, 20g, average	3.8	60

MEAT

OFFAL		FAT(g)	CALS
Brains: lamb, stewed, whole, 85g average		8.0	116
Haggis: 100g, boiled		21.5	308
Heart:	Beef/Ox, 100g, cooked	2.6	148
	Lamb, 100g, cooked	7.9	184
	Veal, 100g, cooked	5.9	189
Kidney:	Beef/Ox, 2, stewed, 100g	2.7	134
	Lamb, 2, stewed, 80g	6.3	147
	Veal, 2, stewed, 90g	6.0	150
Liver:	Beef/Ox/Pig, 100g, stewed/simmered	11.7	221
	Lamb, 100g, fried	13.7	243
	Lamb's Fry & Bacon, 100g	32.8	440
	Veal/calf, 100g, grilled	8.1	188
Sweetbreads: 100g crumbed, fried		14.5	230
Tail: Oxtail/Beef, 100g, stewed/simmered		29.3	351
Tongue:	Beef/Ox, 100g, stewed/simmered	25.1	311
	Lamb, 100g, stewed/simmered	20.4	278
	Lamb, canned (**Tom Piper, Bronte**) 110g can	19.6	250
	Pig, 100g, stewed/simmered	17.5	250
Tripe: 100g, cooked		2.8	83

SMALLGOODS, PROCESSED, COLD & CONTINENTAL MEATS

Many of the highly processed meats, knobs etc. are high in fat. Try to limit your intake - remember that at a party it is very easy to overdose on sliced continental meats!

Average all brands - varied serving sizes	FAT(g)	CALS
Berliner Fleischwurst, 30g	5.5	68
Black Pudding, 30g	5.9	81
Bologna, 30g	5.9	81
Brawn, 50g	8.3	110
Cabanossi, 30g	9.5	109
Camp Pie, tinned, 50g	4.2	78
Chicken Roll, 30g	2.7	46
Corned Beef, tinned, 50g	6.7	108
Corned Beef with Cereal, tinned, **Boston**, 50g	6.2	97
Devon, Chicken Devon, 30g	5.5	71
Devon low fat **Lean Links**, 30g	3.0	48
Fritz, 30g	5.5	75
Garlic knob, 30g	5.7	75
German Beef, 30g	5.2	69

MEAT

SMALLGOODS, PROCESSED, COLD & CONTINENTAL MEATS

Varied Serving Sizes		FAT(g)	CALS
Ham: Off the bone, fresh	Leg, 1 slice, 30g	2.3	42
	Shoulder, 1 slice, 30g	1.8	34
Pressed, Packaged	Leg, 1 slice, 25g	1.3	24
	Shoulder, 1 slice, 25g	1.5	27
Tinned	Deli Ham Light (**Plumrose**), 50g	4.3	70
	Leg, 50g	2.7	57
	Low Fat (**Plumrose Light**), 50g	2.0	54
	Shoulder, 50g	2.9	60
Ham & Chicken Roll, 1 slice, 25g		4.5	58
Hamper, 50g		7.0	109
Kabana, 30g		7.4	85
Lamb's Tongue (**Tom Piper**), 50g		9.8	114
Liverwurst, 20g, 1 Tbsp.		5.8	65
Luncheon Beef, tinned:	**Imperial**, 50g	8.5	112
	Tom Piper reduced salt, 50g	6.0	95
Mortadella, 30g		8.8	98
Pastrami, 30g		5.0	45
Paté: liver, 1 Tbsp., 20g		4.9	60
Margaret's Kitchen, 20g		3.6	45
Plumrose:	tinned leg ham, 50g	2.0	53
	tinned Light Deli Chicken, 50g	4.0	70
	tinned Light Deli Turkey, 50g	4.0	70
	tinned Deli Beef/Deli Ham, 50g	4.0	70
Polish Sausage, 30g		5.3	73
Polony, 30g		6.3	42
Roast Beef, 1 slice, 40g		2.3	60
Silverside, 1 slice, 40g		2.1	60
packaged, 1 slice, 25g		1.3	37
Salami, average all varieties:		11.3	130
Danish, 30g		12.0	135
Hungarian, 30g		11.2	129
Mettwurst, 30g		11.3	130
Milano, 30g		11.1	129
Pepperoni, 30g		10.8	128
Longa Life vegetarian Not Pepperoni, 1 stick, 25g		3.8	68
Polish, 30g		5.3	80
Turkey salami, **Tegel's**, 30g		1.2	34
Spam, 50g serve		15.3	167

MEAT

SMALLGOODS, PROCESSED, COLD & CONTINENTAL MEATS

Varied Serving Sizes	**FAT(g)**	**CALS**
Primo Lite: packaged meats - values given are for 100g. To find the fat and calorie content of each slice divide the figures given by the number of slices in the pack.		
Corned Beef/Leg Ham	3.0	105
Mortadella	20.4	256
Pastrami	4.9	128
Roast Beef	3.0	11
Salami	34.7	398
Shoulder Ham	3.2	103
Strassburg, 30g	5.8	74

Vegetarian: *see **Longa Life & Sanitarium** - Meals packet & canned, page 138.*

MEAT - POULTRY

Poultry is generally low in fat. The amount of fat does vary a little between the various cuts of meat, eg. breast meat has less fat than thigh meat.

Most importantly however, to keep fat levels to the minimum:-

1. ***Do not eat the skin - it contains almost 50% fat!***
2. ***As for beef, lamb etc. only eat the lean portions not the fatty ones!***

CHICKEN

		FAT(g)	CALS
Breast: raw fillets, 100g,	no skin	2.3	111
	skin left on	10.2	172
Dry Roasted/Baked/Microwaved:			
	100g, no skin (cooked weight)	4.8	157
	100g, skin left on (cooked weight)	12.5	215
¼ Roast:	small, no skin, 100g edible	4.8	157
	medium, no skin, 160g edible	7.7	251
	small, skin left on, 100g	12.5	215
	medium, skin left on, 160g	20.0	345
Drumstick, Dry Roasted/Baked/Microwaved			
	average each, no skin	4.6	90
	average each, skin left on	7.2	115
Fried Chicken, Average all pieces, 70g each		15.0	215

(also see Take Away Foods Page 214)

MEAT - POULTRY

CHICKEN		FAT(g)	CALS
Skin, Baked/Roast			
55g skin, approx. ½ medium chicken		26.5	268
Spicy Skin Free, average all brands:			
Breast, 115g		4.0	170
Drumstick, 75g		3.6	115
Thigh, 120g		8.5	160
Wing, 75g		3.0	115
Stuffing, average serve, ¼ cup, 60g		4.5	110
Thigh: raw fillets, 100g,	no skin	5.5	130
	skin left on	13.0	200
Dry Roasted/Baked/Microwaved:			
	100g, no skin (cooked weight)	8.5	140
	100g, skin left on (cooked weight)	15.0	220
¼ Roast, Leg/Thigh, average, skin left on		18.0	265
Wing, Baked/Roast, 1 medium, 35g, skin left on		5.0	80
Fried, 1 medium, 35g, skin left on		10.0	125

STEGGLES CHICKEN 100g serve			
Breast Fillets:	with skin	4.8	129
	without skin	0.8	96
Chicken Maryland,	with skin	14.5	196
Chicken Thighs,	with skin	13.1	182
Chicken Wings,	with skin	11.7	179
Drumsticks,	with skin	5.0	120
Lovely Legs,	without skin	3.9	110
Maryland Fillet:	with skin	8.5	150
	without skin	6.0	131
Thigh Fillets:	with skin	8.1	146
	without skin	6.0	127

CHICKEN SMALLGOODS

INGHAMS, 30g serving, (1 or 2 slices)		
Chicken Breast Supreme	0.8	37
Chicken Buffet	3.4	55
Chicken Pastrami	1.0	41
Chicken Roll	4.4	64
Seasoned Buffet	2.5	1

MEAT - POULTRY

CHICKEN SMALL GOODS		FAT(g)	CALS
STEGGLES, 30g serving, (1 or 2 slices)			
Chicken Breast Roast		0.8	33
Chicken Continental		5.1	71
Chicken Devon Roll		4.8	70
Chicken Roll		3.8	58
Gold Chicken Roll		3.5	56
Gold Chicken Roll Seasoned		3.8	59
Premium Breast		1.1	34
Tenda Chicken Roll		3.8	59

DUCK, GOOSE, HARE

Just like chicken, these meats should also be eaten without the skin - look at the large difference in the figures below.

Roasted Duck:	100g serve, lean meat only	9.5	185
	100g serve, meat & skin	29.0	400
Roasted Goose:	100g serve, lean meat only	20.0	300
	100g serve, meat & skin	40.0	500
Stewed Hare:	150g serve, meat only	12.0	280

TURKEY

Lean turkey is very low in fat and can be used in many recipes instead of chicken if you prefer - or simply with salad or on a sandwich!

Breast, Roasted/Baked/Microwaved			
	100g, without skin	1.5	135
	100g, with skin	6.5	152
Leg/Thigh, Roasted/Baked/Microwaved			
	100g, without skin	4.0	150
	100g, with skin	9.5	190
PLUMROSE, Tinned, Light Turkey, 30g		2.4	42
STEGGLES raw turkey products, 100g			
Self Basting Breast		9.0	180
Turkey Mince		6.8	130
Turkey Sausages		11.2	173
Turkey Stir Fry		5.4	123
Turkey Roast		8.8	156

MEAT - POULTRY

TURKEY	FAT(g)	CALS
STEGGLES Pre-Cooked turkey products, 100g		
Buffet Carve Fillet	2.3	115
Fillet Royale	2.7	121
Oven Roast Breast with Bone	4.0	143
Roast Breast Fillet	3.0	131
Rolled Roast Breast	1.0	97
TEGELS Raw turkey products, 100g		
Easy-Carve Buffe (flavour basted)	8.0	145
Ready to Roast Breast Roll	1.3	102
Turkey Hindquarter (flavour basted)	11.4	168
Whole Turkey (flavour basted)	8.0	147
TEGELS Pre-Cooked turkey products, 100g		
Breast, rolled	2.3	100
Deli-Carve	4.8	120
Oven Roasted Breast Roll	2.1	113
Oven Roasted Buffe: without skin	1.2	102
with skin	4.8	131
Ready to Roast Breast Roll	1.7	118
Smoked Breast Roll	2.2	107
TEGELS Turkey Smallgoods, 30g serve (1 or 2 slices)		
Sliced Turkey Breast	0.9	32
Turkey Hamwich	0.7	30
Turkey Pastrami	0.9	32
Turkey Salami	1.2	34

MILK, MILK DRINKS, SOY MILK

Milk is an excellent source of many valuable nutrients. If you want to cut down on the fat in your diet don't stop drinking milk/milk products - simply change to a lower fat variety.

TIP: *A trick to getting used to the taste of the lower fat milks is to change gradually, ie. Don't immediately change from a full fat product to a skim milk - choose something in between such as Lite White etc.*

MILK		**FAT(g)**	**CALS**
Full Cream, (3.8% fat):	1 Tbsp., 20ml.	0.8	13
	1 glass, 200ml.	8.0	130
	1 cup, 250ml.	9.8	166
Non-Fat or Skim Milk:			
Average all types:	1 Tbsp., 20ml.	0.0	7
	1 cup, 250ml.	0.2	85
Shape (Dairy Farmers), 250ml.		0.3	116
Reduced Fat, 250ml. cup:			
Dairylite Lo		4.0	115
Dairy Choice		3.3	123
Fit 4		2.5	121
Hi-Lo		4.7	139
Light Start		2.5	115
Lite White		3.5	129
Physical		3.5	130
Trim		4.0	115
CONDENSED MILK			
Full Cream, sweetened condensed, **Nestlé:**			
	1 Tbsp., 20ml.	1.8	68
	½ cup, 125ml.	11.5	416
Skim, sweetened condensed, **Carnation:**			
	1 Tbsp., 20ml.	<0.1	55
	½ cup, 125ml.	0.4	338
EVAPORATED MILK			
Full Cream, Bear, Carnation, Ideal:	1 Tbsp., 20ml.	1.6	30
	1 cup, 250ml.	20.0	358
Reduced Fat, eg **Bear:**	1 Tbsp., 20ml.	0.4	20
	1 cup, 250ml.	5.0	245
Skim, eg. **Carnation:**	1 Tbsp., 20ml.	<0.1	15
	1 cup, 250ml.	1.0	190

MILK, MILK DRINKS, SOY MILK

LONGLIFE (UHT), 1 cup, 250ml.	FAT(g)	CALS
Full Cream, average all types	10.0	166
Reduced Fat: eg. **Hi-Lo**	4.7	139
Smart	3.0	124
Skim: eg: **Devondale**	0.3	86
Balance: Lactose Reduced	10.0	166
High Calcium	0.4	116
Paul's Low Lactose	4.0	115
MILK DRINKS - FLAVOURED		
Berri, Very Slim, 300ml. ctn:		
Iced Chocolate/Choc. Honeycomb/Choc. Orange	2.6	183
Iced Coffee/Iced Strawberry	2.6	176
Breaka, (Paul's) 300ml ctn:		
Caramel/Coffee	5.7	200
Chocolate	6.0	204
Vanilla Malt	5.7	197
Breaka UHT, 250ml: Chocolate	5.0	171
Coffee	4.3	165
French Vanilla/Strawberry	4.3	176
Browne's (W.A.):		
Flavoured Milk, 250ml: Banana, Berry	4.3	159
Chocolate	4.5	162
Coffee	4.3	150
Snow	4.3	166
Chill, 220ml: Chocolate	5.5	184
Coffee	4.2	156
Good One, (Dairy Farmers), 300ml ctn:		
Banana & Malt	10.6	278
Carob	10.7	285
Honey & Malt	10.7	284
Lite White, 300ml ctn: Chocolate	4.0	211
Coffee	3.8	203
Mars Milk Snack, 230ml. ctn.	3.3	178
Milkshakes - Thickshakes, average only:		
1 Milkshake with full cream milk, 320ml/340ml	14.0	300
with skim milk	5.0	220
1 Thickshake, 300ml	10.0	275
Moo, average all flavours, 200ml ctn.	3.0	126
Moove, (Dairy Farmers) 300ml. ctn:		
Chocolate	10.7	238
Coffee, Honeycomb, Strawberry	10.5	228

MILK, MILK DRINKS, SOY MILK

MILK DRINKS - FLAVOURED, servings as stated	FAT(g)	CALS
Oak Lite, 300ml: Cappuccino	3.9	144
Chocolate	4.0	141
Vanilla Malt	3.8	156
Oak UHT, 300ml: Chocolate	10.4	233
Coffee	10.4	228
Strawberry	10.4	236
Paul's: Club, 250ml: Chocolate	10.0	208
Coffee	9.3	198
Go-Lite, 300ml., all flavours	0.3	139
Good One, Malt & Honey, 300ml.	10.8	242
Shayks, Chocolate, 250ml.	8.8	212
Toot, 125ml: Chocolate	2.8	84
Strawberry	2.4	79
Egg Nog, flavoured milk, 300ml.	4.8	208
Peter's, Microfreeze Thickshake, 340ml:		
Chocolate	9.2	311
Vanilla Malt	9.2	305
Queensco-Unity, 300ml. ctn:		
CAB	3.9	183
Cruise all flavours	10.5	243
Egg Nog	10.5	252
Jacaranda	3.9	183
Just Lite	0.3	138
Just Natural	9.9	264
Take Five	10.2	228
Slim'n'Slender, 250ml. ctn:		
Rich Chocolate	0.8	196
Tropical Banana	0.8	231
Sustagen: Gold 250ml. ctn.	9.0	280
Lite 250ml. ctn.	5.0	204
Ultra Slim, 250ml. ctn., Swiss Chocolate	4.5	232

***N.B.** Powdered milk drinks eg. cocoa, milo etc. see Drinks Non-Alcoholic page 83.*

POWDERED MILK	FAT(g)	CALS
Full Cream, 4 Tbsp., 30g		
eg. **Devondale, Sunshine**	8.0	145
Low Fat: 4 Tbsp., 30g		
eg. **Devondale**	2.0	115
Skim/Non Fat: 4 Tbsp., 30g		
eg. **Devondale, Carnation, Diploma, Dutch Jug**	0.3	105
Buttermilk, Healtheries, powdered, 30g	2.7	120
N.Z. Goat's Milk, Healtheries, dried, 30g	8.5	158

MILK, MILK DRINKS, SOY MILK

SOY MILK, 1 cup/glass, 250ml	FAT(g)	CALS
Average all brands	8.0	165
Aussie soy milk	7.3	167
Berri: Natural/Vanilla	5.0	179
Soypreme	4.0	179
Becel: Regular	7.0	155
Light	2.3	110
Carnation, powder soymilk, made up 250ml.	4.3	115
Sanitarium So Good: Plain	8.5	155
Lite	1.3	107
Flavoured	8.0	178
So Natural	7.3	155
Soya King	7.9	100
Soylife: Regular	8.5	167
Low fat	2.3	110
Sungold, **(Dairy Farmers)**	9.0	161
Vitasoy: Plain	7.5	163
Vanilla	6.3	208
VARIOUS OTHER MILKS		
Buttermilk: Whole, 250ml.	5.0	130
(**Dairy Farmers** cultured), 250ml.	4.7	124
Reduced Fat, 250ml.	1.5	98
Skim, 250ml.	<0.1	80
Coconut Milk: drained fresh from nut, 100ml	0.0	25
canned, 100ml.	18.0	200
coconut cream, average, 100ml.	20.0	250
Goats Milk: 250ml.	9.0	168
UHT New Zealand goats milk, 250ml.	6.4	111
Rice Milk, Rice Dream:		
Carob, 240ml.	2.5	160
Carob Lite, 240ml.	3.0	150
Original, 240ml.	2.0	120
Vanilla, 240ml.	2.0	130
Vanilla Lite, 240ml.	2.0	120
Sheep Milk, 250ml.	16.5	255
Whey: **Wheylite,** 1 cup, 250ml.	3.0	83
Whey powder, 1 Tbsp., 11g	<0.1	39

NUTS AND SEEDS

Whilst many nuts and seeds are high in nutritional value they are also high in fat. Limit your intake to just a small helping. Once you open a full packet it's hard to stop!

NUTS			FAT(g)	CALS
30g serve, shelled weight				
Almonds:	raw		16.7	180
	sugar coated		5.6	140
	chocolate coated		13.2	170
	roasted, with salt		17.0	188
Beer Nuts, average			15.0	180
Nobby's, 50g pkt.			24.9	309
Brazil, 30g, 8/9 nuts			21.0	205
Cashews:	raw		14.7	174
	roasted		15.4	191
	Planter's:	Dry Roasted, 50g pkt.	23.8	303
		Honey Roasted, 50g pkt.	23.8	295
	Nobby's,	Salted, 50g pkt.	23.8	303
Chestnuts:	raw		0.5	59
	dried		1.2	113
	roasted		13.6	170
	canned, Waterchestnuts, 30g		0.5	15
Coconut:	Coconut ice confectionery, 30g piece		8.8	147
	Cream (from grated coconut meat), 100ml.		20.0	250
	Dessicated/dry - 1 Tbsp., 7g		4.6	45
	- ¼ cup, 20g		13.0	128
	Fresh, 1 small piece - 2cm. x 3cm., 12g		3.3	33
	Milk (grated coconut & water), 100ml.		18.0	200
	Water (drained fresh from coconut), 100ml.		0.0	25
Hazelnuts, 30g			18.4	190
Macadamia Nuts:		raw, (approx. 7 medium), 30g	23.0	220
		Planter's raw, 30g	23.0	227
		roasted in oil	25.0	245
		choc. coated, 3 pieces	21.0	220
Marzipan, (Almond Paste), 30g			5.4	123
Mixed Nuts:	salted, average, 30g		16.6	190
	Nobby's salted mixed nuts, 30g		16.2	191
Nut Spreads, Melrose Naturals:				
Almond, 1 Tbsp., 20g			11.0	115
Cashew, 1 Tbsp., 20g			9.0	105
Hazelnut, 1 Tbsp., 20g			12.5	124

NUTS AND SEEDS

NUTS continued ...		FAT(g)	CALS
Peanuts:	raw (shelled) with skin, 30g	14.1	168
	roasted, 30g	15.0	180
	Dry Roasted **Planter's:** 30g	14.2	182
	50g pkt.	23.7	303
	Planter's low salt: 30g	15.2	187
	50g pkt.	25.3	312
	Planter's Honey Roasted: 30g	14.3	183
	50g pkt.	23.8	305
	Nobby's Satay Flavoured: 30g	15.5	189
	50g pkt.	25.9	315
	Nobby's Spicy Chilli: 30g	15.6	189
	50g pkt.	26.0	315
	Chocolate Coated, 30g	12.5	169
	Sugar Coated, 30g	7.5	120
Pecans, raw, 30g		21.6	212
Pine Nuts, raw, 2 Tbsp., 30g		21.0	210
Pistachios:	shelled, 30g	15.2	168
	unshelled, 30g	8.4	92
Sesame Nut Mix/Planter's: 30g		14.3	179
	50g pkt.	23.3	299
Walnuts:	shelled, 30g	20.8	208
	chopped, ½ cup, 55g	38.1	381

SEEDS

N.B. As for nuts, many seeds are also high in fat - the amounts given below are for only 1 Tablespoon of seeds!

	FAT(g)	CALS
Linseeds, 1 Tbsp., 10g	2.5	45
Lotus, ½ cup, 35g	1.0	116
Pumpkin/Pepitas, dry, 1 Tbsp., 15g	3.0	52
Safflower, dry, 1 Tbsp., 10g	4.0	54
Sesame, dry, 1 Tbsp., 13g	7.2	77
Sesame Paste, 1 Tbsp., 20g	10.0	143
Squash seeds, dry, 1 Tbsp., 15g	7.0	83
Sunflower seeds, dry, 1 Tbsp., 15g	7.7	84
Tahini Paste, 1 Tbsp., 20g	10.0	115
Watermelon Seeds, dry, ¼ cup, 25g	12.0	135

PASTA, SPAGHETTI, NOODLES

PASTA

Pasta itself (all shapes & sizes, including spaghetti) has little or no fat. It is the accompanying sauces and fats that are generally served with the pasta that contribute all the fat! So, eat plenty of pasta, but keep the cream sauces to a minimum.

Note: Dry pasta approximately triples it's weight when cooked:
eg. 100g dry pasta = approx. 300g cooked

TIP: *When eating out at restaurants choose a pasta with a tomato based sauce instead of a cream based one!*

Dry, Uncooked Pasta	**FAT(g)**	**CALS**
Cannelloni Tubes, average, 11g each, dry	0.1	35
Egg Pasta, 100g, dry	1.5	354
Lasagne Sheets, average, 15g each, dry	0.2	50
Spaghetti, 100g, dry	1.8	346
Spinach/Vegetable Pasta, 100g, dry	1.3	360
Wheat Free/Gluten Free, **Freedom Foods**:		
Lasagna, 100g, dry	0.8	342
Garlic & Parsley Pasta, 100g, dry	0.9	368
Spinach, 100g, dry	0.9	356
Tomato & Basil, 100g, dry	0.7	351
White Pasta, 100g, dry	1.1	345
Wholemeal Pasta, 100g, dry	2.2	322

Cooked Pasta, weights given are for pasta after cooking

	FAT(g)	CALS
Egg: all types, 100g	0.6	132
1 cup, approx. 200g	1.2	264
Spaghetti: 100g (white)	0.5	115
1 cup, approx. 140g (white)	0.8	160
wholemeal, 100g	0.9	132
wholemeal, 1 cup, approx. 150g	1.4	198
Spinach/Vegetable: all types, 100g	0.4	131
1 cup, approx. 190g	0.8	249
White: all types, 100g	0.3	120
1 cup, approx. 180g	0.5	216
Wholemeal: all types, 100g	0.8	132
1 cup, approx. 170g	1.4	224

PASTA, SPAGHETTI, NOODLES

FRESH PASTA	FAT(g)	CALS
Average all types		
Fettucine/Tagliatelle:		
Cooked, 150g (1 cup)	1.2	197
Gnocchi: (vegetable)		
Cooked, 220g (1 cup)	4.4	506
Lasagne: with meat, entrée size, 210/220g	13.2	300
large size, 380/400g	24.0	546
with vegetables, entrée size, 210/220g	8.2	220
large size, 380/400g	19.0	466
Ravioli: Meat Filled, 100g, cooked	5.5	140
Spinach & Ricotta, 100g, cooked	3.2	115
Various Brands		
Barberinis, Fresh Beef Lasagne, 300g serve	26.1	510
Latina, Fresh pastas, 100g, cooked weight:		
Plain	0.8	132
Filled	3.4	194
Gnocchi	1.2	144
Egg Free/No Cholesterol	0.6	172
Leggo's, Fresh pastas, estimates only, 100g, cooked weight:		
Agnoletti with Cheese & Spinach	8.4	290
Fettuccine, all varieties	0.7	134
Potato Gnocchi with Cheese	1.2	144
Ravioli with Beef & Chicken	8.4	290
Tortellini (Meat)	8.4	290

NOODLES	FAT(g)	CALS
Egg Noodles, average all brands:		
100g, dry	1.5	350
1 cup cooked, approx. 150g	0.7	165
1 cup fried, approx. 150g	14.0	240
Rice Noodles: 100g, dry	<0.1	357
100g, cooked	<0.1	120
Wholemeal Noodles: 100g, dry	1.8	320
100g, cooked	0.6	110
Fried Noodles (**Changs**) 50g serve	12.5	250
2 Minute Noodles (**Farmland, Maggi, Trident**), 80g pkt.	15.0	385

PASTRY

Most pastries are high in fat, whether they are sweet or savoury varieties. Limit your intake where possible.

TIP: *When cooking pastry at home use Filo Pastry, because it has only 1.4g of fat per 100g (you can now buy Filo Pastry in chilled packets that will last about 3 weeks in the refrigerator!).*

Instead of spreading each layer with a lot of oil or butter simply spray every second or third sheet with a little Pure and Simple oil spray. Put your favourite low fat filling inside and bake for ½ hour. Makes a great low fat treat!

PASTRY - VARIOUS TYPES, Raw/Unbaked	FAT(g)	CALS
Biscuit Base, 100g	23.0	520
Choux, 100g, raw	15.5	250
Filo Pampas, Frozen: 1 sheet, 16.7g	0.3	51
5 sheets, 83.5g	1.3	256
Pampas, Chilled, 100g	1.6	307
Antoniou, 100g	1.4	308
Flaky, 100g	38.0	390
Packet Pastry:		
Bakeo: Regular, 100g made up	20.0	449
Flaky, 100g made up	36.7	556
Pizza Bases: **Pampas** frozen, 330g each	22.0	914
Farmland fresh, 330g each	5.6	924
Tip Top fresh mini bases, 75g each	1.8	182
Puff: Block, 100g	18.3	354
Roll, 100g	18.3	354
Sheet, 167g each	30.5	591
Butter, each sheet, 188g each	34.4	666
Shortcrust: Block, 100g	21.7	384
Sheet, 180g each	39.0	689
Shortcrust Sweet, 100g	23.3	443
Spring Roll Pastry, Pampas, 1 sheet, 12.5g each	0.3	39
Tart Cases, Pampas: Small, 23g each	5.5	105
Large, 220g each	52.6	984
Wholemeal: 1 sheet, 150g	31.2	530
100g	20.8	354
Vol-au-Vents/Oyster Cases, unfilled:		
Small, 5g each	1.9	28
Medium, 60mm., 12.5g each	4.8	69
Large, 100mm., 25g each	9.7	139

PIZZA - FROZEN

Meat varieties of pizza are the highest in fat (cabanossi, pepperoni etc). Choose small servings or slices and eat slowly. Try making your own pizzas at home - the whole family will love them - see the recipe tip below.

TIP: *Make your own tasty low fat pizza using either pita bread or Pizza Bases (eg. Tip Top), spread with tomato base such as Dolmio, add some grated low fat cheese (eg. Devondale Seven). Top with either left over cold meats, onions, mushrooms or other vegetables or even Soy Feast Vegeburgers then add a little extra cheese and bake in a hot oven for 15-20 mins.*

AVERAGE	**FAT(g)**	**CALS**
1 Whole Pizza Large, 500g	42.0	1100
2 small slices, 125g	10.5	275
McCAIN		
Regular, (500g whole):		
Cheese & Bacon, 125g, 2 slices	12.5	292
Ham & Pineapple, 125g, 2 slices	9.4	273
Supreme, 125g, 2 slices	8.5	279
5 Minute Pizza, ½ whole, 135g (270g whole), Supreme	7.7	285
Pizza Pockets, (400g whole):		
Ham & Pineapple, 100g, (¼)	7.9	237
Pepperoni, 100g, (¼)	11.1	248
Supreme, 100g, (¼)	9.3	245
Pizza Singles, 100g each:		
Cheese & Bacon	8.4	222
Ham & Pineapple	7.5	211
Supreme	7.8	209
Pizza Slice, (600g whole):		
Ham & Pineapple, 150g, 2 slices, (¼)	7.8	322
Supreme, 150g, 2 slices, (¼)	7.7	312
PAPA GUISEPPE		
Regular, (500g whole):		
Cheese & Bacon, 125g, 2 slices, (¼)	9.6	284
Cheese & Tomato, 125g, 2 slices, (¼)	9.9	305
Ham & Pineapple, 125g, 2 slices, (¼)	8.0	284
Supreme, 125g, 2 slices, (¼)	10.5	290
Pizza For One, 100g each: Cheese & Bacon	7.5	249
Ham & Pineapple	5.9	232
Supreme	8.0	251
Party Pizzas, 34g each, Cheese & Bacon	2.3	74

Also see Take-Away and Fast Foods section for other Pizzas, page 218.

PROTEIN POWDERS, DIET SHAKES, MEAL REPLACERS

Many of these products can provide a convenient, nutritious and low fat alternative to a regular light meal such as lunch.

TIP: *Combine 1 or 2 servings of fruit with your meal replacer drink, either eaten separately or blended together.*

AUSSIE BODIES	**FAT(g)**	**CALS**
Energy Extender: Chocolate, 30g dry	0.9	120
Vanilla, 30g dry	0.9	120
Trim Food Meal Replacer, all Flavours, 30g dry	0.5	100
Trim Pancake Meal Replacer, 40g serve	1.0	130
DIET SHAKE		
Made as Directed with 200ml. skim milk:		
Banana Tropicana	0.3	166
Cappuccino	0.5	167
Chocolate	0.7	168
LEAN & FIT		
Meal Replacer Shake, all flavours, 58g dry	3.0	220
LIMMITS, Meal Replacers, each pkt. or meal		
Apricot Almond (2 pieces)	13.0	281
Cheese'n'Chives (4 pieces)	17.5	300
Cheese'n'Oatbran (3 pieces)	16.5	291
Choc. Hazelnut Oat (2 pieces)	17.0	289
Choc. Nut Crunch (2 pieces)	15.0	282
Herb & Chicken (3 pieces)	18.0	299
Mint choc. Slice (3 pieces)	20.0	318
Sultana Munch (2 pieces)	13.5	275
MASSIVE (Nutra Life)		
Amino MCT Growth Fuel, 50g dry	5.0	201
High Protein Muscle Builder, 75g dry	0.7	110
Heavy Duty Weight Gainer, 75g dry	11.9	313
Low Fat Rapid Gainer, 100g dry	0.5	364
Maximum Protein 90%, 30g dry	0.1	110
Muscle Builder, 30g dry	0.2	116
Super Pro Weight Gainer, 50g dry	6.1	211
Super Pro Vegetable Protein Weight Gainer, 50g dry	6.0	210
Ultra Low Fat Maxigain, 81g dry	0.1	300

PROTEIN POWDERS, DIET SHAKES, MEAL REPLACERS

MUSASHI	FAT(g)	CALS
Slim Food, average all types, 30g dry	0.4	80
NUTRA-FIBRE		
Diet Shake, average all flavours, 31g dry	0.2	110
NUTRA LIFE		
Amino Carb, 33g dry	0.0	122
Carboplex, 31g dry	0.0	118
Milk & Egg, 30g dry	1.4	126
NUTRA TRIM		
Diet Shake, 33g dry	0.7	355
PETER McCARTHY 'BALANCE'		
Pro-Sport Protein Drink, average all flavours, 375ml. ctn.	1.1	282
TRIM		
Diet Shake, 40g dry	1.0	145
ULTRA SLIM		
Banana Smoothie, made with skim milk, 200ml.	0.3	167
Meal Replacer Shakes, made as directed with		
200ml. of skim milk: Cappuccino	0.6	171
Chocolate	0.8	174
Strawberry	0.4	171
Vanilla	0.6	173
WEIDER		
Dynamic Carbo Energiser, 60g dry	0.0	224
Firmaloss Shake, 20g dry	0.0	71
Victory: Body Cuts, 65g dry	1.0	120
Body Mass, 65g dry	1.0	250
Carbo Fire, 65g dry	0.0	237
Lean'n'Hard Rapid Gainer, 100g dry	0.8	362
Mega Mass 2000, 90g dry	<0.1	324
WEIGHT WATCHERS		
Shake Mixes, average all flavours, 30g dry	<1.0	100

RESTAURANTS - ETHNIC CUISINE

This section should be used only as a guide to the fat and calorie values of the meals listed. Obviously there will be large variations from one restaurant to another. Some restaurants may even offer to modify a special dish for you if you request it. However, often this luxury will not be available. Remember, when you do eat out try to choose wisely from the menu (avoid all fried foods) but don't forget to enjoy yourself! (Don't forget your Fat Budget - you can always spread it out over a few days!).

Where a serving size is given, again this is only an estimation - you may need to adjust the figures up or down depending on whether you eat a larger or smaller serve than that shown.

ASIAN

Best choices here include steamed rice, vegetable or combination type dishes. Sweet & Sour dishes whilst low in fat are often high in calories.

250g serve unless stated differently		**FAT(g)**	**CALS**
Baak Choy (Chinese Cabbage) with Oyster Sauce, 200g		10.0	180
Beef & Black Bean Sauce		18.0	290
Beef Chow Mein		22.0	360
Beef Curry (Thai Muslim with coconut milk)		44.0	620
Beef in Oyster Sauce		24.0	375
Beef Satay		25.0	440
Beef Teriyaki		19.0	450
Chicken Braised in B.B.Q. Sauce		18.0	310
Chicken Chop Suey		17.0	300
Chicken Chow Mein with Noodles		28.0	415
Chicken with Cashews or Almonds		25.0	350
Crisp Fried Chicken with Lemon Sauce		29.0	490
Crisp Skin Chicken, deep fried		35.0	510
Combination Chow Mein		24.0	370
Curried Prawns with Rice		14.0	270
Curry Puffs (Thai), meat filled:	Large, 85g each	30.0	350
	Mini, 30g each	11.0	125
Curry with Coconut Milk (Thai), average, all types		42.0	600
Dim Sims, deep fried:	Regular, 50g each	4.5	110
	Mini, 17g each	1.5	40
Duck, deep fried with lemon/orange sauce		40.0	565
Roast Duck, 200g (incl. skin), with spicy sauce		60.0	720
Fried Rice, 1 cup (175g)		11.0	320
Gow Chees		11.0	125
Ham & Chicken Roll, 175g		15.0	480
Ice Cream Balls, deep fried, each		13.0	175

RESTAURANTS - ETHNIC CUISINE

ASIAN continued..	FAT(g)	CALS
Long Soup, 1 bowl	3.5	130
Lychees, 6 fresh, (60g)	0.1	40
Noodles, 1 cup, fried, 100g	11.5	155
Noodles, Thai, 100g	20.0	285
Pork Braised with Vegetables	22.0	400
Pork with Plum Sauce	50.0	580
BBQ Pork in Special Sauce	38.0	595
Pork Ribs in Black Bean Sauce	36.0	500
Pork - Sweet & Sour	24.0	450
Prawn & Coconut Curry	21.0	350
Prawn Chow Mein	28.0	365
Prawn Cutlets, each	4.0	65
Prawn Omelette	28.7	463
Garlic Prawns (entrée, 175g)	16.0	220
King Prawns battered & fried, in honey sauce	36.0	600
Prawns in Satay Sauce	22.0	355
Prawns - Sweet & Sour Sauce	11.0	300
Rice: Fried, 1 cup	11.0	320
Steamed/Boiled, 1 cup	0.5	240
Short Soup, 1 bowl	7.8	235
Spring Rolls, each	5.0	115
Sweet & Sour Sauce, 1 Tbsp.	0.0	24
Vegetable Stir Fry	10.0	180
Wontons fried, 30g	9.8	115

GREEK

Often based around vegetables, many Greek dishes are quite low in fat.

Serving size as listed		
Baklava (honey topped filo pastry with nut filling) 1 pastry	18.0	245
Cabbage Rolls, 150g each	6.0	185
Calamari (Squid) crumbed & deep fried, 100g (approx. 8-10 rings)	9.5	205
Dolmathakia Latheres (stuffed vine leaves) 4 small, served with yoghurt	6.0	150
Domestica (Greek Wine), 1 glass	0.0	100
Feta Cheese, 30g	7.0	84
Fried Eggplant in batter, 100g	10.0	120
Galactaboureko (custard filled pastry), each	14.0	342
Halvas (nut dessert), 100g	12.9	212

GREEK continued ...	FAT(g)	CALS
Kataifi (Pastry soaked in honey & nuts), each	12.4	380
Loukoumathes (small honey puffs), each	2.0	50
Moussaka: entrée 150g	14.4	228
main 300g	29.0	560
Octopus (squid) BBQ'D with sauce, 200g	6.0	275
Olives, black - 6 medium	6.4	40
Pastitso (Macaroni & Meat Pie), 300g	38.5	690
Retsina (Greek Wine), 1 glass	0.0	100
Souvlakia, each	6.8	120
Spanakopita (Cheese & Spinach in Filo), each	22.2	318
Stifatho (Casserole: Lamb, Potato & Onion), 250g	16.5	320
Stuffed Tomatoes (Meat & Rice), 125g each	7.5	125
Taramosalata (Fish roe dip), 1 Tbsp., 25g	5.0	60
Tiropitakia (Cheese & Egg Traingles in Filo), 100g	25.0	358
Tzatziki (Cucumber, Garlic & Yoghurt Dip), 1 Tbsp., 25g	3.0	33

INDIAN

Many Indian dishes provide a reasonably low fat meal. Watch the inclusion of yoghurt in sauces and keep fried foods to a minimum.

Serving size as listed		
Beef Curry, 250g	16.5	344
Beef Kofta (Meatball) Curry, 200g	35.0	520
Beef Vindaloo, 250g	16.0	440
Brinjal Bartha (Eggplant Purée), ¼ cup	8.0	100
Chapati (wholemeal bread rounds), each	2.0	60
Chicken Curry, 250g	20.0	410
Chicken Pilau, 200g	23.0	550
Chicken Tandoori, ¼ chicken	21.0	394
Chatni Dhania (Coriander Chutney), 1 Tbsp.	<0.1	20
Chatni Podina (Ground Mint Chutney), 1 Tbsp.	<0.1	20
Cucumber Salad with sour cream, side dish serve	7.5	90
Curry Puffs (meat filled), 30g	11.0	125
Dhal, ½ cup	3.0	105
Fish Curry, 250g	14.0	330
Lamb Curry, 250g	15.0	336
Lamb & Potato Curry, 250g	15.0	400
Braised Lamb & Yoghurt, 250g	20.0	466
Lamb Kebabs, each skewer	6.0	135
Lamb Kofta (Meatballs) in Yoghurt Sauce, 200g	40.0	580

RESTAURANTS - ETHNIC CUISINE

INDIAN continued..	FAT(g)	CALS
Mixed Vegetable Bhaji (Spicy fried veg), 250g	25.0	292
Mulligatawny Soup, 1 bowl	16.0	275
Pakorhas (Savoury vegetable fritters), each	9.0	150
Parathas (Flaky wholemeal bread), each	15.0	230
Pappadams, 1 large: fried	2.5	50
grilled or microwaved	0.0	25
Pork Vindaloo, 250g	28.0	600
Puris (deep fried bread rounds) 18cm, round, each	7.0	120
Ras Gulas (Balls of cream cheese in syrup), each	6.0	200
Rotis (Ceylonese version of Chapatis but with the addition of coconut), each round	6.0	105
Samoosas (small meat filled pastries), 40g each	11.0	150
Singaras (small vegetable filled pastries), 40g each	10.0	140

N.B. For Indian Sauces etc. eg. Pataks, Sharwoods, see Sauces on page 192

ITALIAN

Many Italian meals are based on pasta which contains virtually no fat. It is the sauces that accompany the pasta that can contain a lot of fat. Avoid cream or cheese based sauces - instead choose tomato or vegetable based ones. Also watch your serving size. Italian meals tend to be rather large!

Serving size as listed	FAT(g)	CALS
Antipasto: varies greatly - average each meat slice	11.0	135
Calamari, crumbed & deep fried, 100g (8-10 rings)	9.5	205
Cassata, 1/8 20cm. round	29.0	425
Chicken Cacciatore, 300g	8.5	285
Chicken Marsala, 300g	24.0	650
Florentines, small, each	7.5	160
Gelato, 2 scoops	0.0	72
Lasagne: Meat - entrée, 220g	13.2	300
- main course, 400g	24.0	546
Spinach/Vegetable - entrée, 220g	8.2	220
- main course, 400g	19.0	466
Minestrone Soup, 1 bowl (varies with amount of oil used in cooking)	12.5	240
Mussell Soup, 1 bowl	5.8	240
Osso Bucco, 300g	28.8	575

RESTAURANTS - ETHNIC CUISINE

ITALIAN, continued...		FAT(g)	CALS
Pasta: Plain, cooked, 1 cup approx. 140g		0.8	160
Including Linguine, Fettuccine, Macaroni, Penne, Spaghetti, Tagliatelle etc.			
With the following sauces:			
Bolognese:	entrée, 220g	10.0	330
	main course, 400g	18.0	600
Carbonara:	entrée, 220g	23.0	400
	main course, 400g	42.5	725
Marinara (no added cream):	entrée, 220g	8.0	320
	main course, 400g	14.4	575
Napolitana:	entrée, 220g	6.6	255
	main course, 400g	12.0	460
Pesto:	entrée, 220g	15.0	330
	main course, 400g	27.2	600
Alfredo:	entrée, 220g	39.8	555
	main course, 400g	70.0	995
Pizza: ¼ of a 30cm. round pizza, average only			
Cheese & Tomato		14.0	330
Ham & Pineapple		11.0	305
Pepperoni/Cabanossi		20.0	400
Seafood		12.0	315
Supreme		14.0	350
N.B. Also see Frozen Pizza page 172 and Take Away foods page 218.			
Polenta, 60g		1.5	206
fried pieces, each		7.5	270
Potato Gnocchi (potato dumplings), 200g		5.2	165
with Bolognese sauce, 220g		14.0	310
Ravioli/Tortellini, with meat, 200g		11.0	270
Ravioli with Ricotta & Spinach, 200g		6.5	224
Scallopine (Veal with wine & cream), 250g		14.5	410
Siena Cake, 1 slice, 60g		10.0	200
Spaghetti, *see Pasta above*			
Stuffed Tomatoes, each		5.0	135
Tortellini with Cream Sauce, 250g		38.0	650
Zabaglione (marsala dessert), 1 serve		6.5	170

N.B. For Italian sauces etc. see Sauces page 190.

RESTAURANTS - ETHNIC CUISINE

LEBANESE

Many Lebanese dishes, like Greek dishes, are based around vegetables. Dips etc. will vary depending on the amount of oil used. Generally you should try to only eat small amounts of these tasty dips.

Serving size as listed	FAT(g)	CALS
Baba Ghannouj (Sesame & Eggplant Dip), 1 Tbsp., 25g	5.0	60
Baklava (honey topped filo pastry with nut filling), 1 pastry	18.0	245
Cabbage Rolls, 150g each	6.0	185
Falafel, 2 patties	8.0	125
Abundant Earth falafel mix, 100g	4.5	360
Foule Moudamass (Broad Beans), 60g	1.6	44
Hommus (puree from chick peas), 1/3 cup	17.1	226
Kafta, 2	10.2	165
Kebbi (meat, wheat & pinenuts), 125g	8.9	225
Lebanese Bread, 1 round	2.3	276
Lady Fingers, 2 pastries	14.6	239
Shish Kebab (lamb kebabs), 1 skewer	6.6	124
Spinach Pie, 100g	20.6	290
Tabbouleh, ½ cup	12.6	145
Turkish Delight, square	0.0	50
Vine Leaves, rice filled, 4 small	4.5	130

MEXICAN & SPANISH

Many Mexican & Spanish meals are based on bread type foods such as tacos, tortillas & burritos. The main sources of fat in Mexican & Spanish meals comes from the added cheese or sour cream sauces. Choose bean fillings over meat and avoid the guacamole and corn chips! Salsa is a low fat alternative.

Serve size as listed		FAT(g)	CALS
Burrito:	Bean, 1 only	11.0	310
	Beef or Chicken, 1 only	16.0	370
Chilli Con Carne:	Beans only, 250g	3.0	220
	Beans & meat, 250g	8.0	300
Corn Chips, 100g *(See snack foods page 200)*		34.0	556
Enchilada:	Bean, 1 only	9.0	270
	Beef or Chicken, 1 only	14.0	310
Guacamole (Avocado Dip), ¼ cup		24.0	250
Huevos Rancheros	(eggs baked with tomatoes chillies) 1 serve = 2 eggs	20.0	325
Mexican Style Rice, 1 cup, 170g		0.3	160

RESTAURANTS - ETHNIC CUISINE

MEXICAN & SPANISH continued...			FAT(g)	CALS
Nachos,	with beans:	entrée, 200g	19.0	415
		main course, 350g	33.0	725
	with beef/chicken:	entrée, 200g	25.0	500
		main course, 350g	43.0	875
Paella:	Chicken, 300g		20.0	500
	Seafood, 300g		17.0	450
Quesados, avocado & sour cream,				
1/8 15cm. round tortilla, (hors d'oevres size)			3.5	57
Refried Beans 'Frijoles Refritos', 100g			0.8	81
Sangria, 1 glass			0.0	120
Taco: beef, bean or chicken, 1 only			15.0	240
Tortilla, 15cm. round, 1			0.5	60
Tortilla Pizza with beef & cheese, 15cm. round			25.0	410
Tostado (fried tortilla), no topping			4.0	85
Tostado:	with Beef & Beans, 1 only		16.0	320
	with Chicken, 1 only		14.0	280
Torta de Cielo (traditional almond sponge cake),				
1/8 of 20cm. round cake - plain			10.5	250
	- with 2 Tbsp. whipped cream		18.5	325

N.B. *Also see Meals - canned & packet for other Mexican foods eg. Casa Fiesta & Old El Paso.*

RICE, RICE CAKES, RICE DISHES

Rice is a nutritious low fat food - include plenty of it in your everyday diet.

RICE			FAT(g)	CALS
	Brown Rice/Wild Rice:	½ cup, raw, 100g	2.6	364
		1 cup, boiled, 180g	1.7	275
	Sungold (parboiled):	½ cup, raw, 100g	1.4	354
		1 cup, boiled, 175g	0.7	220
	White Rice:	all varieties:		
		½ cup, raw, 100g	0.5	357
		1 cup, boiled, approx. 175-180g	0.4	220
		1 cup, fried, approx. 170-180g	8.0	310
RICEBRAN				
	Sunfarm:	1 Tbsp., 8g	1.6	32
		½ cup, 55g	11.0	241

N.B. See Breakfast Cereals (page 33 for rice based cereals.)

RICE CAKES				
	Average all brands, 1 cake, 12.5g		0.4	44
	Carob Coated:	1 regular size, 50g	14.0	250
		1 small size, 35g	9.5	170
RICE DISHES				
	Paella, 250g		17.0	450
	Pilaf, 250g serve		4.0	200
	Rice Pudding, *see Dairy Desserts Page 44*			
	Risotto, 250g		9.0	280
RICE FROZEN				
	Logan Farm:	Pre-Cooked Natural, 50g	0.0	183
		Pre-Cooked Brown & Wild Rice, 50g	1.0	186

SALADS - FRESH & TINNED

Salads purchased from retail outlets will obviously vary greatly in their fat and calorie contents, so use the list below as a general guide. Always feel free to ask the retailer what type of dressing has been used if you are unsure and remember 'Cholesterol Free' does not mean Fat Free!!

TIP: *To keep fat content down in salads, choose either a low fat dressing or a vinegar/lemon/garlic style of dressing. As the old saying goes 'Hold the Mayo!' (In other words, don't add the mayonnaise!).*

FRESH	**FAT(g)**	**CALS**
Food Outlets etc, estimates only:		
Bean Salad, 1 cup, 200g	5.0	250
Caesar Salad, 1 cup, 200g	22.0	300
Coleslaw, 1 cup, 190g	10.0	200
Niçoise Salad, 100g	6.5	190
Pasta/Macaroni Salad, 1 cup, 250g	15.0	350
Potato Salad: with mayonnaise, 1 cup, 200g	24.0	350
with low fat yoghurt, 1 cup	3.0	280
Rice Salad, 1 cup, 190g	8.0	280
Spinach & Sesame Salad, 1 cup, 150g	8.0	100
Tabouli, ½ cup, 110g	12.6	145
Waldorf, 1 cup, 200g	24.0	360
TINNED		
Heinz Garden Bean Salad, 100g	1.4	80
Hawaiian, 100g	4.9	117
Potato Salad, 100g	4.7	93
Traditional Vegetable Salad, 100g	3.3	71
Masterfoods, 100g		
Beans'n'Corn	1.2	97
Mixed Beans	0.9	54
Mixed Vegetables	0.2	44
Potato Salad	6.6	115
Rice Salad	0.2	72
Tropical Salad	0.1	86
Zucchini Salad	0.6	41

SALAD DRESSINGS

***TIP:** Look for oil free or no oil dressings & remember that a label that reads Low Cholesterol or No Cholesterol does not mean Low Fat!*

COLESLAW DRESSINGS 1 Tbsp., 20g		**FAT(g)**	**CALS**
Average all brands:	Regular	6.0	79
	Reduced Fat	2.0	30
Eta, regular		3.4	55
Kraft:	Regular	7.0	85
	Light	1.1	11
	Free	2.2	41
Praise:	Classic/Canola	6.9	80
	Light	3.7	56
	Salad Magic	2.3	51

FRENCH DRESSINGS 1 Tbsp., 20g		**FAT(g)**	**CALS**
Average all brands:	Regular	5.0	53
	Reduced Fat	<0.1	4
Kraft:	Regular	4.4	49
	Light	0.0	7
	Free	0.0	8
	French & Herb Free	0.0	5
	Olive Oil Classics	4.0	42
	French Herb & Garlic	5.4	54
Masterfoods, French Vinaigrette		5.7	66
No Frills (Franklins), Regular		4.0	43
Praise:	Regular	3.6	41
	No Oil	0.0	11
Salad Magic, French with Garlic, No Oil		<1.0	8
Weight Watchers, singles, each		0.0	6

ITALIAN DRESSINGS 1 Tbsp., 20g		**FAT(g)**	**CALS**
Average all brands:	Regular	6.5	62
	Reduced Fat	0.0	6
Kraft:	Regular	6.0	59
	Light	0.0	1
	Free	0.0	4
	Olive Oil Classics	6.0	59
Masterfoods, Italian Vinaigrette		5.7	54
No Frills (Franklins), Regular		4.0	43
Praise:	Regular	3.6	38
	No Oil	0.0	8
Salad Magic		<1.0	13
Weight Watchers, singles, each		0.0	4

SALAD DRESSINGS

MAYONNAISE 1 Tbsp., 20g		FAT(g)	CALS
Average all brands	Regular, 1 Tbsp., 20g	6.5	75
	Reduced Fat, 1 Tbsp., 20g	4.0	57
	90% Fat Free, 1 Tbsp., 20g	2.0	34
Eta, mayonnaise		3.2	47
Freedom Foods, Egg Free, No Cholesterol		4.2	65
Gold'n'Canola		3.1	49
Heinz		7.0	72
Kraft:	Natural	5.5	67
	Light	2.4	41
	Free	1.8	34
	Miracle Whip	10.2	100
Masterfoods, Squeeze On		2.9	39
Norganic, Soya Mayonnaise		11.6	105
Praise:	No Cholesterol	7.0	75
	Light	3.0	47
	Low Oil	5.5	70
Weight Watchers		1.9	35

THOUSAND ISLAND DRESSING 1 Tbsp., 20g		FAT(g)	CALS
Average all brands:	Regular	4.5	52
	Reduced Fat	2.0	33
Kraft:	Regular	7.0	76
	Light	2.3	36
	Free	2.0	33
Masterfoods, Squeeze On		6.3	72
No Frills (Franklins), Regular		4.8	60
Salad Magic, Regular		2.2	44

VARIOUS MISCELLANEOUS DRESSINGS & BRANDS		FAT(g)	CALS
Eta, Potato Salad Dressing		4.2	50
Kraft:	Creamy Caesar	6.8	70
	Miracle Whip	10.2	100
	Original Style Potato Salad Dressing	7.0	73
	Tartare Sauce Regular	6.0	65
	Tartare Sauce Homestyle	5.0	55
Masterfoods:	Seafood Cocktail	2.4	40
	Tartare	12.8	115
Praise:	Coconut Curry	7.3	78
	Basil/Thai/Peppercorn/Tomato with Basil & Oregano	7.0	78
	Sour Cream & Chives	7.6	82
Salad Magic:	Spicy Thai	0.0	12
	Herb & Garlic	<1.0	9
	Sour Cream & Chives	2.3	49
	Tropical Hawaiian	0.0	18

SANDWICHES

The values given for the sandwiches listed below are based on 2 average size slices of bread (any kind) with 1 teaspoon of butter or margarine plus an average size serving of the filling used (unless stated differently).

TIP. *To minimise your fat intake avoid using any butter or margarine. You would then need to adjust all of the following figures by SUBTRACTING 4.0g of fat and 36 calories from the values given.*

Similarly if you use 2 teaspoons of butter or margarine instead of only 1 teaspoon then you will need to ADD another 4.0g of fat and 36 calories to the figures below.

	FAT(g)	CALS
Asparagus & Cheese (1 slice)	15.5	310
Avocado (½ small)	23.5	350
Bacon (1 rasher)	15.5	320
Bacon & Grilled Cheese (1 slice)	25.5	440
Bacon & Grilled Cheese Croissant	50.0	680
Bacon & Egg	21.0	275
Baked Beans	6.0	225
Banana	5.5	250
Cheese (1 slice) & Tomato	15.5	310
Cheese (1 slice) & Salad	15.5	325
Cheese (1 slice) & Vegemite	15.5	300
Chicken (50g)	10.5	275
Chicken (50g) & Avocado	28.5	450
Chicken & Avocado Croissant	52.0	670
Chicken (50g) & Salad	10.5	300
Chicken & Salad Croissant	28.0	500
Corned Beef & Lettuce	10.5	265
Corned Beef & Tomato	10.5	275
Curried Egg	10.5	250
Devon & Tomato	14.5	325
Egg	10.5	250
Egg & Lettuce	10.5	255
Egg & Prawns	11.5	300
Egg & Tomato	10.5	265
Egg & Salad	10.5	275
Gherkin & Cottage Cheese	6.6	220
Ham (50g)	9.5	254
Ham & Cheese (1 slice)	19.5	395
Ham, Cheese & Tomato	19.5	410
Ham, Grilled Cheese & Tomato Croissant	44.0	650
Ham & Tomato	9.5	275

SANDWICHES

	FAT(g)	CALS
Mortadella	14.5	280
Peanut Butter (1 Tbsp.)	15.5	300
Prawn & Avocado (½ small avocado, 50g prawns)	24.5	400
Prawns & Mayonnaise (50g prawns)	9.0	255
Rissole & Tomato Sauce	20.5	515
Roast Beef (50g)	10.5	265
Roast Beef Roll/Hot	18.5	395
Roast Beef & Lettuce	10.5	270
Roast Lamb & Mint Jelly	11.0	275
Roast Lamb Roll/Hot	19.0	400
Salad	5.5	220
Salami (30g all types average)	16.7	305
Salmon	9.0	260
Salmon & Salad	9.0	280
Sausage (1 only) & Tomato Sauce	18.5	370
Smoked Salmon	8.0	245
Spaghetti	5.8	215
Turkey (Roast, 50g) & Cranberry Sauce	9.0	280
Turkey & Salad	9.0	285
Tuna (50g)	7.0	235
Tuna & Cheese (1 slice)	17.0	355
Vegemite	5.5	180

Different Breads & Additional Fillings
ADD the following figures....

		FAT(g)	CALS
Bread Roll instead of sliced bread:	Round	0.0	0
	Long roll	1.0	50
Pita Bread instead of sliced bread:	Small	0.0	0
	Large	0.5	50
Toasted Sandwiches:	(both sides buttered!)	4.0	40
	still only one side buttered	0.0	0
Cream Cheese, 1 Tbsp., 20g		7.9	84
Lettuce		0.0	5
Mayonnaise,	1 tsp., 5g	2.5	30
	1 Tbsp., 20g	6.5	75
Mustard, 1 tsp., 5g		0.1	4
Pickles/Chutney/Relishes, average, 1 Tbsp.		0.0	35
Salad (Lettuce, Tomato, Cucumber, Beetroot etc.)		0.0	30
Salt, Pepper		0.0	0
Thousand Island Dressing:	1 tsp., 5g	1.2	15
	1 Tbsp., 20g	4.5	52
Tomato Sauce, 1 Tbsp.		0.0	15

SANDWICH SPREADS - TOAST TOPPERS

Choose from the many low fat spreads available - try using them without any butter.

TIP: *If you cannot go without butter or margarine - make sure you spread it very thinly - just a scrape.*

		FAT(g)	CALS
Butter/Margarine:	regular spread, 1 tsp., 5g	4.0	36
	reduced fat	2.0	18
Cheese Spread, Kraft:	regular, 1 Tbsp., 20g	5.0	60
	light, 1 Tbsp., 20g	3.3	48
Cream Cheese Spread, average all brands:			
	1 Tbsp., 20g	7.0	70
	Kraft Light, 1 Tbsp., 20g	4.5	57
Chocolate Spreads, 1 rounded tsp., 8g		3.0	45
Fish Pastes/Spreads:			
	Average all brands, 1 tsp., 5g	0.5	9
	John West, Tuna Spread, 1tsp., 5g	0.6	10
	Kraft, ave. all flavours, 1 tsp., 5g	0.5	10
	Masterfoods, average all flavours, 1 tsp.	0.5	9
	Pecks, Anchovette/Salmon & Shrimp, 1 tsp., 5g	0.3	6
Freedom Foods, Sugar Free Spreads, 1 tsp., 6g		0.0	10
Fruit Spreads, Average all types:			
	1 Tbsp., 25g	0.0	40
Golden Syrup/Treacle:	1 tsp., 6g	0.0	19
	1 Tbsp., 25g	0.0	80
Honey, average all types:	1 tsp., 6.5g	0.0	20
	1 Tbsp., 25g	0.0	80
Jam/Marmalade, average all types:	1 tsp., 5g	0.0	16
	1 Tbsp., 25g	0.0	65
	¼ cup, 80g	0.0	208
Low Joule/Diet varieties eg **Cottees, Weight Watchers**:			
	1 tsp.	0.0	2
	1 Tbsp., 25g	0.0	7
Lemon Butter Spread, average all brands:			
	1 tsp., 6.5g	0.4	18
	1 Tbsp., 25g	1.6	72
	Home made, 1 tsp., 7g	1.0	70

SANDWICH SPREADS - TOAST TOPPERS

	FAT(g)	CALS
Meat Pastes/Spreads:		
Average all brands, 1 tsp., 5g	0.5	9
Kraft, average all flavours 1 tsp., 5g	0.5	9
Masterfoods: Corn'n'Bacon, 1 tsp., 5g	0.3	5
Devilled Ham & Chicken	0.5	9
Other flavours, 1 tsp., 5g	0.9	10
Pecks: Chicken, Chicken & Ham, 1 tsp., 5g	0.8	10
Devilled Ham, 1 tsp., 5g	0.6	9
Pepperoni, Veal, Ham & Chicken, 1 tsp., 5g	0.6	8
Nut Spreads:		
Melrose 'Naturals': Almond Spread, 1 Tbsp., 20g	11.0	115
Hazelnut Spread, 1 Tbsp., 20g	12.5	124
Cashew Spread, 1 Tbsp., 20g	9.0	105
Nutella, 1 tsp., 8g	3.0	40
Paté, average all types, 1 Tbsp., 20g	4.9	60
Peanut Butter: average all brands, 1 Tbsp., 20g	10.0	127
no added salt, 1 Tbsp., 20g	10.0	119
Kraft: Crunchy/Smooth, 1 Tbsp., 20g	10.3	127
No added salt, 1 Tbsp., 20g	10.3	119
Sanitarium: all types, average 1 Tbsp., 20g	10.0	141
Promite, 1 tsp., 6g	<0.1	10
Sandwich Spread/Kraft, 1 Tbsp., 20g	1.0	30
Sesame Paste, 1 Tbsp., 20g	10.0	143
Tahini Paste, 1 Tbsp., 20g	9.6	115
Vegemite/Marmite, 1 tsp., 6g	0.0	6

SAUCES & CONDIMENTS

SAUCES - GENERAL	FAT(g)	CALS
Average all brands		
Aioli Sauce, 1 Tbsp., 20g	16.0	145
Apple Sauce, 1 Tbsp., 20g	0.0	17
Alfredo Sauce, ½ cup	45.0	452
Bar-B-Q Sauce, 1 Tbsp., 20g	0.0	35
Kraft Homestyle, 1 Tbsp., 20g	0.0	13
Bearnaise, 1 Tbsp.	9.0	85
Bechamel, 1 Tbsp., 20g	5.0	55
Beef & Black Bean Sauce, ½ cup	1.0	65
Bolognese, ½ cup	15.0	200
Butterscotch, ½ cup	32.0	230
Caramel Sauce, ¼ cup	19.0	310
Carbonara Sauce, ½ cup	35.0	386
Cheese Sauce: (packet mix) average, ½ cup.	5.0	120
homemade, ½ cup	21.0	260
Chilli Sauce, 1 Tbsp.	0.1	12
Cranberry Sauce, 1 Tbsp.	0.0	30
Custard, ½ cup	5.0	110
Gravox, 1 Tbsp. powder	0.0	27
Gravy, made up, ½ cup	0.5	36
Horseradish, raw, 1 tsp., 6g	0.0	4
Horseradish cream (**Masterfoods**), 1 tsp.	0.7	11
Marinara, no cream, ½ cup	3.0	140
Mint Sauce, 2 tsps.	0.0	10
Mint Jelly (**Masterfoods**) 1 Tbsp., 20g	0.0	50
Mustard, ave. all types, 1 tsp.	0.1	4
Onion Sauce (from packet), ½ cup	1.0	35
Oyster Sauce, 1 Tbsp., 20g	0.0	15
Parsley Sauce (from packet), ½ cup	5.0	120
Pesto, ¼ cup	45.0	414
Rich Neapolitan, ½ cup	5.0	130
Rich Sicilian, ½ cup	6.5	146
Salsa, 1 Tbsp.	0.0	10
Satay, ¼ cup, (homemade)	13.0	160
commercial, 1 Tbsp., 20g	2.2	55
Soy Sauce, 1 Tbsp.	0.0	14
Spicy Plum/Vegetable, 1 Tbsp., 20g	0.0	15
Spicy Red, 1 Tbsp., 20g	0.0	14
Steak Sauce, 1 Tbsp., 20g	0.0	30
Sweet'n'Sour, ½ cup	0.0	130
Kraft, Homestyle Sweet'n'Sour, 1 Tbsp., 20g	0.0	13

SAUCES & CONDIMENTS

SAUCES - GENERAL		FAT(g)	CALS
Taco Sauce, 1 Tbsp., 20g		0.5	15
Tartare Sauce, 1 Tbsp., 20g		5.5	60
Tomato Sauce: 1 Tbsp.		0.0	22
	¼ cup	0.0	135
White Sauce (from packet), ½ cup		11.0	175
Worcestershire Sauce, 1 Tbsp., 20g		0.0	14
Vinegar, 1 Tbsp., all types		0.0	3
TOMATO SAUCES, PASTES, PURÉE			
Tomato Sauce, average all brands, 1 Tbsp.		0.0	22
Weight Watchers, 1 Tbsp.		0.0	13
Tomato Paste, average all brands: 1 Tbsp., 26g		<0.1	16
	100g	0.5	60
Leggo's:	Plain, 140g ctn.	1.2	140
	With Basil & Oregano, 100g	0.5	67
	With Garlic & Herbs, 100g	0.6	69
	With Onions & Herbs, 100g	0.6	83
	With Wine & Chilli, 100g	0.5	62
Tomato Purée average all brands: 100g		0.3	30
	Edgell: 425g can	1.3	136
	Leggo's: 425g can	1.7	195
Tomato Relish average 1 Tbsp., 20g		<0.1	20
Heinz Tomato Combo, average all varieties, 435g can		6.0	174
CONDIMENTS			
Chutney; average all brands, 1 Tbsp., 22g		<0.1	40
Rosella low Joule Chutney, 1 Tbsp.		<0.1	10
Corn Relish (**Masterfoods**), 1 Tbsp., 20g		<0.1	17
Cucumber, pickled, dill pickle, 1 large, 100g		<0.1	15
Gherkin, pickled, 1 medium, 25g		<0.1	5
Gherkin Relish (**Masterfoods**), 1 Tbsp., 20g		<0.1	30
Masterfoods Farmhouse Relish, 1 Tbsp., 20g		<0.1	29
Mustard, average all types, 1 tsp., 5g		-0.1	4
Mustard Relish (**Masterfoods**), 1 Tbsp., 20g		<0.1	17
Sweet Mustard Pickles (**Leggo's**), 1 Tbsp., 20g		<0.1	21
	(**Masterfoods**), 1 Tbsp., 20g	<0.1	15
Olives:	Green, 1 medium, 6g	0.2	2
	Black, 1 medium, 6g	1.0	8
	Stuffed, 6 medium, 50g	4.3	45
Onions, pickled:	1 small, 10g	0.0	3
	1 large, 20g	0.0	7
Pickles Low Joule (**Rosella**), 1 Tbsp., 20g		<0.1	6

CONDIMENTS continued...		FAT (g)	CALS
Salsa, average all brands, all types, 1 Tbsp., 20g		<0.1	10
Masterfoods, 1 Tbsp., 20g:	Chilli	0.5	9
	Mild	0.5	8
	Spicy	0.5	8
Sandwich Relish **Kraft,** 1 Tbsp., 20g		1.0	30
Tomato Relish/Pickles, 1 Tbsp., 20g		<0.1	19
Uncle Ben's Spicy Salsa Casserole, 1 Tbsp.		0.1	1

PACKET, CANNED, BOTTLED - VARIOUS BRANDS

CAMPBELL'S

	FAT (g)	CALS
Real Sauces, Undiluted, 100ml.		
Beef & Red Wine	1.0	43
Chicken & Herb Gravy	2.5	50
Diane Sauce	4.0	67
Pepper Sauce	3.4	58

CONTINENTAL

	FAT (g)	CALS
Cup-a-Sauce, ¼ packet, 60ml. (made as directed):		
Cheese	1.9	50
Curry	1.2	46
Mushroom	1.4	38
Pepper	0.5	31
Plum	0.4	45
Satay	2.6	55
Steak Diane	0.6	36
White	1.8	48
Gravy: Brown Onion Gravy, 1 pkt.	2.3	121
Roast Meat Gravy, 1 pkt.	2.5	120
Perfection Meat Coatings, whole packet:		
Honey & Sesame Chicken	5.9	233
Spicy Chinese Chicken	0.8	167
Continental/Rosella Hot Pot Casserole Base		
Packet contents **only**, whole packet, dry:		
Creamy Mornay	16.2	530
Curry	4.1	461
French Onion	3.4	313
Mushroom	10.1	336
Savoury	5.1	342
Sweet & Sour	3.6	530
Tomato Provencal (Rich Tomato)	3.1	312

SAUCES & CONDIMENTS

PACKET, CANNED, BOTTLED - VARIOUS BRANDS		FAT(g)	CALS
FREEDOM FOODS			
Sugar Free Sauces, 1 Tbsp., 20g:	Barbeque	0.1	13
	Mild Chilli	1.8	20
	Tomato Chutney	<0.1	14
	Tomato Sauce	0.1	6
HOLBROOK'S			
Chicken Dippin':	Mango'n'Apricot, 100g	0.0	177
	Rich & Tangy Marinade, 100g	0.8	125
Satay Stir Fry:	100g	6.6	156
	1 Tbsp., 20g	1.3	31
Stir Fry:	100g	2.7	153
	1 Tbsp., 20g	0.5	31
KRAFT 1 Tbsp., 20g			
Homestyle BBQ & Onion		0.0	16
Homestyle Sweet & Sour		0.0	17
Homestyle Tartare		5.0	55
Tartare		6.0	65
(also see Salad Dressings, page 184)			
LATINA 100g serve			
Carbonara		12.2	169
Creamy Bacon & Mushroom		13.4	160
Hot Siciliana		2.6	65
Meat Bolognese		2.9	80
LAWRY'S			
Cook in Sauce, 100g			
Cantonese		0.3	108
French		4.0	61
Hungarian Goulash		2.9	84
Indian		1.4	42
Mexican		0.5	38
Russian		9.7	109
Spanish		3.9	68
Thai		6.3	102
Marinade Mixes, 1 pkt. (dry ingredients only)			
Beef		0.5	84
Chicken		0.8	88

PACKET, CANNED, BOTTLED - VARIOUS BRANDS	FAT(g)	CALS
LAWRY'S continued...		
Packet Sauces, each pkt. (dry mix only - you must add any extra milk or butter/margarine used to make up. ***TIP**: Delete any butter altogether and use skim milk*).		
Bearnaise	2.9	122
Beef Burgundy	1.0	98
Hollandaise	4.6	136
Mornay	1.6	122
Pepper Steak	0.5	146
Rich & Thick Pasta Sauce	1.8	148
Spaghetti	0.7	153
Steak Diane	0.2	146
LEGGO'S		
Concentrated Pasta Sauce, 100g serve:		
Olive Pesto	15.7	203
Sundried Tomato Pesto	17.6	228
Traditional Basil Pesto	27.2	318
Italian Cooking Sauce, 100g serve:		
Bolognese with Garlic & Onions	0.3	59
Bolognese with Mild Chilli	0.5	67
Chunky Napolitana	0.8	63
Chunky Garden Vegetable	0.5	62
Chunky Tomato, Onion & Garlic	0.4	53
Rich Tomato	0.5	65
Rossini Style with Capsicum	0.2	41
Spaghetti Sauce: with Beef, ½ can 220g (440g can)	8.8	165
with Bacon, ½ can 220g (440g can)	6.4	142
Weekday Goumet, 250g serve:		
Chinese Sweet & Sour	0.5	167
Creamy Wine & Mushrooms	27.0	319
Indonesian Satay	19.3	316
Mild Indian Curry	9.0	193
Parmigiana	2.5	123
MAGGI		
Packet Sauce Mixes, ¼ packet, made as directed:		
Brown Onion	1.5	25
Cheese	2.9	54
Chicken	0.6	18
Diane	0.8	22

SAUCES & CONDIMENTS

PACKET, CANNED, BOTTLED - VARIOUS BRANDS	FAT(g)	CALS
MAGGI Packet Sauces continued...		
Green Pepper	0.8	36
Mint	0.7	20
Parsley	2.0	46
Parsley with skim milk	0.7	34
Rich Meat	0.6	18
Satay	5.0	89
Sweet & Sour	0.3	52
White	2.0	45
White with skim milk	0.8	34
MASTERFOODS		
Cuisine Essentials, 1 Tbsp., 20g:		
Chinese	0.4	29
Indian	0.9	20
Italian	0.3	15
Mexican	0.6	18
Thai	0.1	11
Dolmio Chunky, 100g serve:		
Capsicum & Chilli	0.5	52
Eggplant, Capsicum & Shallots	0.6	50
Farmhouse Vegetables	0.3	57
Garden Vegetables	0.2	46
Olive & Mushrooms	1.6	64
Onion & Mushrooms	0.5	48
Tomato, Onion & Garlic	0.2	43
Dolmio Provinciale, 100g serve:		
Chicken Cacciatore	0.4	49
Creamy Carbonara	8.3	121
Creamy Mushroom	8.0	104
Italian Cooking Sauce	0.3	30
Seafood Marinara	0.4	50
Veal Parmigiana	2.0	69
Vegetarian Tomato & Herb	1.3	35
Vegetarian Olive & Chilli	2.6	54
Dolmio Traditional, 100g serve:		
Capsicum/Mushroom	0.4	48
Spicy Peppers/Tomato & Basil	0.6	50
Tomato	0.4	39

SAUCES & CONDIMENTS

PACKET, CANNED, BOTTLED - VARIOUS BRANDS	FAT(g)	CALS
MASTERFOODS continued...		
Kan-Tong, 250g serve:		
Black Bean	3.0	127
Honey Sesame & Garlic	1.5	83
Lemon	0.3	142
Mongolian Lamb	5.3	184
Spicy Plum	1.0	187
Spicy Sweet'n'Sour	0.5	261
Sweet'n'Sour	0.5	261
Sweet'n'Sour Lite	0.5	174
Thai Sweet'n'Sour	1.5	142
Stir Fry Sauces, 115g serve:		
Sesame & Teriyaki	3.0	113
Soy & Garlic	0.0	55
Sweet & Sour	0.7	205
Sweet Chilli & Lime	0.3	204
McCORMICK		
Classic Packet Sauce Mixes, 1 pkt., dry ingredients only:		
Bearnaise	0.2	111
Green Peppercorn	4.5	127
Hollandaise	5.9	89
Mushroom	4.6	157
Gravy Mixes, 1 pkt., dry ingredients only:		
Chicken Gravy	0.8	67
Chicken Gravy Lite	0.1	65
Country Herb Gravy	0.1	84
English Mint Gravy	2.2	86
Lite Rich Sauce Gravy	0.2	66
Onion & Mushroom Gravy	1.2	69
Rich Brown Gravy	1.3	72
Marinades, 1 pkt., dry ingredients only:		
Beef	1.1	99
Packet Sauce Mixes, 1 pkt., dry ingredients only:		
Chicken Cacciatore	0.5	144
Cheese Sauce	4.8	130
Parsley White Sauce	3.9	118
Peppersteak	3.0	137
Steak Diane	6.8	160
Tuna Casserole	0.5	122
Tuna Mornay	9.4	179

SAUCES & CONDIMENTS

PACKET/CANNED/BOTTLED - VARIOUS BRANDS		FAT(g)	CALS
McCORMICK'S			
Pasta Sauces, 1 pkt., dry ingredients only:			
	Bolognese	0.3	133
	Carbonara	7.1	147
	Creamy Seafood	2.0	98
	Herb & Garlic	2.7	55
Seasoning Mixes, 1 pkt., dry ingredients only:			
	Beef Rice	0.9	76
	Chicken Rice	0.5	68
	Chinese Style Rice	2.1	60
	Hamburger Mince	0.5	121
	Indian Style Rice	1.9	82
	Italian Style Rice	5.0	116
	Savoury Mince	0.6	119
	Spanish Style Rice	0.8	105
	Stir Fry	0.3	110
	Thai Rice	2.3	101
OLD EL PASO *(also see Page 144)*			
Nachos Topping, 100g		<0.1	67
Seasoning Mixes:	Burrito, 100g pkt.	2.6	322
	Chilli, 35g pkt.	1.6	100
	Taco, 35g pkt	1.0	93
Taco Sauce, all types, 100g		<0.1	31
Thick & Chunky Salsa, all types, 100g		<0.1	27
PATAKS Indian Sauces			
Jars, 100g serve:	Daplazi, mild	3.1	94
	Jalfrezi, mild sweet	4.9	122
Tinned, 100g serve:	Delhi, Mild	13.1	155
	Korma, Medium	9.5	142
	Madras, Hot	19.8	219
	Moglai, Medium	7.8	111
	Rogan Josh, Medium	10.7	133
	Tikka Marsal, Medium	13.3	170
	Vindaloo, Hot	24.0	258

SAUCES & CONDIMENTS

PACKET, CANNED, BOTTLED - VARIOUS BRANDS		FAT(g)	CALS
RAGULETTO			
100% Natural, ¼ jar, 125g (500g jar):			
Basilico		<1.0	45
Bolognese		1.2	67
Calabrese		<1.0	50
Capri		<1.0	56
Florentine		<1.0	43
Napolitana		1.6	64
Parmigiana		<1.0	46
Romano		1.9	62
Sicilian		<1.0	58
Venetian		1.7	70
Gourmet Range, ⅓ jar, 125g, (375g jar):			
Arrabiata, 125g		9.4	79
Boscaiola, 120g, (360g jar)		9.5	119
Carbonara, 120g, (360g jar)		11.3	136
Mediterranean, 125g		5.5	105
ROSELLA			
Chicken Tonight, 125g serve:			
Apricot		0.7	69
Cacciatore		2.4	72
Creamy Peppercorn, 120g serve		9.3	118
Curried Chicken, 120g serve		1.7	45
French		12.4	134
Herb & Wine		6.3	91
Lemon		10.5	132
Mushroom		11.0	124
Oriental		1.1	66
Spicy Salsa		0.3	48
Sweet & Sour		<1.0	140
SHARWOOD'S			
Indian Sauces, Tinned, 100g serve:	Curry do Piazza	5.0	95
	Tandoori Markhani	5.7	88
Balti Stir Fry Curry Sauces, 100g serve (430g jar):			
Joshani		2.5	53
Kesari		5.6	79
Shahee		6.5	89
Indian Madras Vegetable Curry, 100g serve (270g jar)		5.5	87
Indian Korma Vegetable Curry, 100g serve (270g jar)		6.7	101
Indian Rajmah Vegetable Curry, 100g serve (270g jar)		3.3	82

SAUCES & CONDIMENTS

PACKET, CANNED, BOTTLED - VARIOUS BRANDS	FAT(g)	CALS
UNCLE BEN'S		
Simmer Sauces, ¼ jar, 125g, (500g jar):		
Apricot Chicken	0.4	73
Beef Strogonoff	5.6	97
Creamy Chicken & Mushroom	8.8	131
Devilled Sausage	0.4	57
Hawaiian Sweet & Sour	0.2	120
Hungarian Goulash	0.5	63
Mild Chicken Curry	8.4	117
Savoury Mince	1.7	65
Savoury Steak	1.5	73
Tuna Mornay	5.9	90
WEIGHT WATCHERS		
Pasta Sauce, ½ cup, 125g	<1.0	47

SNACK FOODS - POTATO CRISPS, PRETZELS, POPCORN ETC.

Most snack foods are high in fat, salt and calories, even when consumed in small amounts. Try to snack on low fat foods such as fresh fruit or even dried fruit - save these high fat snacks for the occasional indulgences!

***TIP**: Oven baked pretzels are a good low fat choice!*

	FAT(g)	CALS
Bagel Crisps, average all flavours, 30g serve	4.0	130
Bradsnax: Dhall, 50g serve	10.1	231
Honey Sesame Fingers, 50g serve	16.4	263
Indian Pakoda, 50g serve	18.6	275
Pea Snacks, 50g serve	15.4	260
Satay Nibbles, 50g serve	13.3	247
Burger Rings: - 50g serve	13.2	250
- 21g serve (multipacks)	5.5	105
Cheetos: Cheese & Bacon Balls - 50g serve	17.0	266
- 21g serve	7.1	120
Cheese Burgers - 50g serve	17.4	263
- 21g serve	7.3	111
Cheese Things - 50g serve	18.6	272
- 21g serve	7.8	114
Cheezels: Cheese - 50g serve	15.4	260
- 21g serve	6.5	109
Cheese & Bacon - 50g serve	16.8	268
- 21g serve	71.0	113
Cheez-Ums (Pringles): 50g serve	18.5	295
190g carton	70.3	1119
Cheese Snacks:		
Cheeseana Snack Pack, 30g serve	7.1	111
Dippity Bics: Pineapple & Ham, 25g serve	5.8	95
Other flavours, 25g serve	7.0	102
Uncle Toby's Le Snak, Ave. all flavours, 25g serve	5.3	83
Chick Pea Chips (Freedom Foods) low salt, 50g serve	18.0	272
Chick Pea Crisps (Freedom Foods) low salt, 50g serve	15.1	257
Corn Chips: CC's, average all flavours - 50g serve	12.8	250
- 21g serve	5.4	105
Doritos: Plain Toasted - 50g serve	9.6	214
Spicy Nachos - 50g serve	11.7	208
Tasty Cheese - 50g serve	10.9	228
- 25g serve	6.0	105
Freedom Foods, low salt - 50g serve	9.5	214

Corn Chips continued...	**FAT(g)**	**CALS**
Muncheros: Cheese - 65g serve	21.9	342
Golden Corn - 65g serve	22.8	348
Lime & Chilli - 65g serve	21.3	340
Tostitos (Tortilla Chips) - 50g serve	15.0	263
Firecrackers (Planters): 50g serve	14.5	257
250g packet	72.3	1285
Fruit & Nut Mix, average all brands, 50g serve	9.0	190
Fruit & Nut Mix - Tropical, average all brands, 50g serve	10.0	205
Fruit & Nut Snacks (Mellow Yellow), 50g serve:		
Brunch Mix	8.0	144
Cashew Delight	13.5	218
Fruit & Almond	8.5	204
Fruit Nut & Seed	12.0	207
Fruit Salad Chunks	<1.0	124
Nature Mix	14.0	221
Nibble Mix	11.5	185
Raw Nut Deluxe	22.5	166
Roasted Unsalted Nuts	23.0	223
Fruit Snacks:		
Bellis - Fruit Bars, 20g each, average	1.0	75
Freedom Foods - Fruit Strips, average 20g each	0.0	44
Sun Valley True Fruits - Fruit Bars, 20g each:		
Apple/Pear, average	<0.1	52
Other flavours, average	<0.1	44
Uncle Toby's - Fruit Snacks, 25g serve	5.7	117
- Roll Ups, average, each	1.0	57
Golden Dippers (Planters), 50g serve	4.5	113
Health Snack Foods, *see page 116*		
House of Treats - snack buns/cookies, each:		
Anzac Cookie, 85g	24.0	413
Anzac Slice, 85g	24.0	413
Chocolate Topped Anzac, 60g	17.0	301
Choc.Chip Cookie, 85g	20.0	408
Choc.Chip Round Cake, 85g	21.0	399
(also see Health buns, cookies etc. page 116)		
K & S, 50g serve:		
Murkoo Spicy Crisps	15.0	257
Papri (Chick Pea Crisps)	18.0	272

SNACK FOODS: POTATO CRISPS, PRETZELS, POPCORN ETC.

	FAT(g)	CALS
Mellow Yellow Snack Mixes, 50g serve:		
Apricot Coconut Slice	2.6	183
Apricot Delight	2.6	183
Bhuja Mix	15.0	253
Bombay Chips	10.5	230
Carob Buttons	15.5	263
Licorice	<0.1	167
Licorice Carob Twists	1.3	183
Mixed Bhuja (Tixana), 50g serve	15.0	235
Muesli Bars, *see page 116*		
Noodle Snacks (Mamee), 50g serve	8.5	224
Oriental Mix (Tixana), 50g serve	15.0	235
Pappadums (Planters), 25g serve	6.9	122
Pasta Whirls (Planters), 50g serve	10.7	232
Popcorn: Commercial, oil popped, 1 cup, 8g	2	40
Green's Poppin, 100g pkt.	8.0	349
Home prepared, air popped (no oil), 1 cup, 8g	0.3	27
Movie Theatre, 1 medium bucket, 25-30g	6.5	125
Sugar Coated, average all types, 30g	1.2	130
Uncle Toby's: Lite, ¼ 100g pkt.	3.7	95
Microwave, ¼ 100g pkt.	7.4	116
Pork Rind Snacks, 25g serve	7.0	122
Potato Crisps/Chips:		
Average all brands including Arnott's, Frito-Lay, Freedom Foods, Lay's, Ruffles, Samboy, Smith's, Tixana.		
Plain/Flavoured: 25g serve	8.5	135
50g serve	17.0	270
21g serve (multipack)	7.1	114
Kettle Chips:		
Hawkers - Honey Baked Ham, 50g serve	17.6	280
Lay's, Hawkers - average, 50g serve	19.0	360
Smith's - slow cooked potato, 50g serve	14.0	250
slow cooked Chilli Flav., 50g serve	13.4	244
Pringles, average all flavours: 50g serve	18.8	280
190g carton	71.0	1080
Pringles Light, all flavours: 50g serve	12.6	256
170g carton	42.5	870
Smith's Lites (lightly salted): 50g serve	16.0	260
21g serve (multipack)	6.7	110

SNACK FOODS: POTATO CRISPS, PRETZELS, POPCORN ETC.

	FAT(g)	CALS
Prawn Crackers, 25g serve	5.5	117
Pretzels: Average all brands & shapes, 50g serve	3.5	189
Lay's Bavarian Twists, 50g serve	3.5	194
Tiny Twists, 50g serve	2.5	194
Parkers Oven Baked		
wheat sticks, twists, 50g serve	1.5	193
Pizza Minis, 50g, serve	6.0	216
Rice Crackers, Average all brands, 50g serve	9.0	220
Smax: Cheese flavour, 50g serve	11.6	245
Vegetable Flavour, 50g serve	9.3	232
Seashells Marinara (Planters), 50g serve	12.2	239
Snackwell Peaz, 50g serve	13.2	230
Soya Crisps/Chips (Tixana): Crisps, 50g serve	13.5	233
Chips, 50g serve	15.0	239
Space Food Sticks (White Wings):		
Caramel, per twin stick	2.5	73
Chocolate, per twin stick	2.8	71
Straws/French Fries, (Smith's), 50g serve	15.0	255
Toobs, Tasty, 50g serve	9.5	215
Twisties: Cheese, 50g serve	13.2	249
Chicken, 50g serve	12.4	247
Tangy BBQ, 50g serve	16.2	265
Tomato Tang, 50g serve	15.4	260
Vege-Chips, average all flavours, 50g serve	13.0	248

SOUPS - PACKET & CANNED

Soups can be a very nutritious, low fat inclusion in your everyday diet. Whether they are homemade, packet or canned - try to eat soups that do not contain cream and when adding milk to canned soups use a low fat or skim milk instead of whole milk.

To calculate the fat and calorie content of homemade soups, simply measure out all the ingredients and add up their respective fat and calorie values to find out the total value of your soup.Then divide these totals by the number of servings of soup to find out how much fat and how many calories are in one bowl of soup!

CAMPBELLS	FAT(g)	CALS
All Natural ¼ can, 220g, made as directed, (440g can):		
Garden Mushroom	4.6	75
Garden Pea	2.9	103
Garden Tomato	0.4	62
Garden Vegetable	1.8	79
Spicy Tomato	0.2	62
Tomato & Vegetable	0.9	55
All Natural Creamy, ¼ can, 220g, made as directed, (440g can):		
Asparagus	13.0	172
Carrot	5.5	120
Corn	5.9	128
Potato & Leek	13.9	189
Pumpkin	4.2	103
Smoked Salmon	8.4	139
Sweet Potato	8.8	167
Chunky, ½ can, undiluted, 220g (440g can):		
Beef	6.8	174
Beef & Mushroom	2.6	110
Beef & Pasta	4.0	141
Chicken, Chicken & Pasta	3.1	132
Ham & Pea	4.8	174
Lamb	7.5	169
Minestrone	2.9	136
Potato & Bacon	11.9	224
Stockpot	3.7	134
Vegetable	1.3	101
Condensed, ¼ can, made as directed, 220g (440g can):		
Beef Consomme, Chicken Consomme	0.1	24
Chicken Vegetable	2.2	64
Country Vegetable	1.1	55
Italian Tomato	0.2	55
Old Fashioned Stockpot	0.7	70

SOUPS - PACKET & CANNED

CAMPBELLS	FAT(g)	CALS
Condensed continued...		
Split Pea with Ham	2.9	147
Tomato	0.2	55
Vegetable	0.7	68
Vegetable Beef	0.7	101
Cream Of, ¼ can, made as directed, 220g (440g can):		
Asparagus	6.2	147
Broccoli & Cheese	7.3	117
Celery	6.8	119
Chicken	7.0	125
Chicken & Corn	5.1	119
Chicken & Mushroom	9.9	150
Mushroom	7.9	136
Mushroom & Bacon	6.8	117
Pumpkin	5.9	150
CONTINENTAL		
Cup-A-Soup, 1 pkt. made as directed, 200ml. cup:		
Chicken Noodle	1.0	42
Chicken Noodle salt reduced	0.8	39
Chicken & Vegetable	0.6	59
Chinese Chicken & Sweet Corn	1.0	67
Country Chicken & Onion	1.6	64
Cream of Celery	3.2	83
Cream of Chicken	2.5	86
Cream of Mushroom	2.8	88
Creamy Corn	2.2	77
Garden Potato & Leek	1.2	68
Hearty Beef & salt reduced	0.5	56
Hot & Spicy Tomato	0.5	69
Pea & Ham	1.5	84
Singaporean Golden Vegetable	1.7	73
Spring Vegetable	0.2	38
Tomato	1.0	81
Cup-A-Soup Special, 1 pkt. made as directed, 250ml. cup:		
American Creamy Potato & Ham	3.4	126
Chicken & Corn with Croutons	4.1	138
Creamed Pumpkin with Croutons	3.3	123
Creamed Vegetable	8.1	161
Creamy Lemon Chicken with Rice	5.0	144
Creamy Pumpkin with Croutons	3.3	123
Creamy Sweet Potato with Croutons	3.3	131

SOUPS - PACKET & CANNED

CONTINENTAL	FAT(g)	CALS
Cup-A-Soup Special, continued...		
Dutch Curry & Rice	3.0	110
French Creamy Mushroom & Wine	5.0	130
Hearty Chicken	5.2	129
Malaysian Spicy Chicken	4.9	130
Seafood Bisque	5.5	150
Spanish Tomato with Croutons	1.5	112
Vegetable & Beef	3.1	115
Virginia Pea & Ham	2.6	126
Lots of Noodles, made as directed, 200ml. serve:		
BBQ Beef	0.5	119
BBQ Chicken	1.0	101
Beef	1.3	122
Chicken	1.4	128
Chinese Golden Chicken & Corn	4.6	151
Country Tomato & Corn	1.8	118
Cream of Chicken	3.2	130
Creamy Chicken Satay	1.9	117
Mild Curry	2.7	125
Tomato	1.4	127
Vegetable	1.1	113
Packet Soups, made as directed, 250ml. (¼):		
American Creamy Corn	0.5	44
Bacon & Onion	0.8	44
Cheese & Leek	1.3	65
Chicken Noodle	0.6	48
Chicken Noodle salt reduced	0.5	47
Chinese Vegetable	0.4	35
Cream of Chicken/and salt reduced	0.9	52
Cream of Mushroom/and salt reduced	0.7	54
Cream of Onion	2.6	78
Dutch Curry & Rice/and salt reduced	1.0	71
French Onion/and salt reduced	0.1	34
Hearty Beef	1.4	68
Hungarian Beef Goulash	0.8	44
Indian Mild Curry	0.8	47
Italian Tomato with Oregano & Basil	0.4	52
Minestrone	0.4	58
Thick Vegetable/and salt reduced	0.3	57
Savoury Chicken Supreme	2.0	67
Savoury Tomato with Noodles	1.3	81
Seasoned Chicken & Vegetable	1.1	56

SOUPS - PACKET & CANNED

CONTINENTAL	FAT(g)	CALS
Packet Soups continued...		
Spring Vegetable	0.2	26
Tomato	0.6	75
Tomato & Vegetable	0.9	58
Slim-A-Soup, 1 sachet, made as directed, 200ml.		
Chicken Primavera	1.6	47
Chicken Noodle	0.6	29
Chicken with Wholemeal Croutons	2.0	39
Creamy Cheese & Cauliflower	0.9	50
Curried Harvest Vegetable	1.0	52
Garden Broccoli	1.2	42
Garden Vegetable	0.3	34
Mild Malay Chicken Curry	0.9	39
Mushroom & Chives	1.5	39
Pea & Ham Supreme	1.3	57
Pumpkin & Vegetable	0.3	34
Tomato & Herb	0.3	38
FARMLAND		
Quick Cup, 1 sachet, made up, 200ml.		
Chicken & Vegetable	<1.0	56
Chicken Noodle	1.0	38
Cream of Chicken	2.5	69
Cream of Mushroom	2.1	67
Cream of Pumpkin	1.5	61
Hearty Beef	<1.0	54
Pea & Ham	1.1	70
Tomato	<1.0	69
HEINZ		
All Natural, ¼ can, 220g, made as directed, (440g can):		
Creamy Carrot	4.0	99
Creamy Mushroom	6.8	119
Creamy Pumpkin	6.8	150
Creamy Sweet Corn	6.8	143
Tomato & Basil	0.2	77
Veal & Rice	3.7	86
Chunky Pot'o'Soup: ½ can, 220g, undiluted, (440g can):		
Beef Pepperpot	2.4	165
Beef with Vegetables	2.9	128
Chicken	8.1	163
Chicken & Corn	4.2	119

HEINZ	FAT(g)	CALS
Chunky Pot'o'Soup, continued...		
Ham & Pea	3.1	93
Spring Lamb	9.0	220
Tomato Tortellini	0.7	130
Veal & Bacon	8.6	204
Classics, ¼ can, 220g, made as directed, (440g can):		
Creamy Asparagus & Leek	7.3	154
Creamy Chicken Supreme	10.8	176
Creamy Pumpkin & Leek	7.5	152
Creamy Seafood Bisque	12.1	211
Condensed: ¼ can, 220g, made as directed, (440g can)		
Beef Barley Broth	2.2	73
Beef Paprika	0.9	59
Chicken & Vegetable	0.4	55
Creamy Asparagus	8.1	132
Creamy Celery	9.0	145
Creamy Chicken	9.9	161
Creamy Chicken & Asparagus	6.4	121
Creamy Chicken & Corn	7.3	132
Creamy Chicken & Mushroom	8.6	136
Creamy Mushroom	9.0	147
Creamy Potato & Leek	7.3	130
Creamy Pumpkin	7.5	136
Creamy Seafood	8.8	136
Dinosaurs in Tomato	0.7	88
Italian Style Chicken	0.9	92
Minestrone	1.5	62
Mulligatawny	1.8	75
Pea & Ham	1.8	108
Tomato / and salt reduced	0.9	66
Tomato & Bacon	1.8	77
Vegetable	1.1	71
Vegetable Beef	2.2	82
Zesty Tomato	1.1	75
Soup for One, 220g can, undiluted:		
Beef & Vegetable	2.9	88
Chicken Noodle	0.9	82
Creamy Chicken	8.4	134
Creamy Pumpkin	7.1	130
Creamy Tomato	5.7	128
Minestrone	0.9	95

SOUPS - PACKET & CANNED

HOUSE OF WINSTON	FAT(g)	CALS
Fresh Soups, 225g serve:		
Carrot with Orange & Coriander	<0.1	47
Celery with Stilton Cheese	1.7	73
Pumpkin with Coriander & Ginger	<0.1	51
Tuscan Bean Soup	1.6	116

P. M. U.

¼ can, 220g, made as directed, (440g can):		
Chicken & Vegetable	1.1	46
Cream of Chicken	1.5	44
Cream of Mushroom	1.3	55
Pea & Ham	1.5	101
Spring Vegetable	0.4	40
Tomato	1.1	64
Tomato & Bacon	1.8	79
Vegetable Beef	1.5	64

ROSELLA

¼ can, 220g, made as directed, (440g can)		
Beef Goulash	2.8	78
Chicken & Corn	2.4	70
Chicken & Rice	1.8	90
Chicken & Vegetable	1.5	53
Cream of Chicken	4.8	84
Cream of Chicken salt reduced	4.0	82
Cream of Mushroom	5.3	86
Farmhouse Vegetable	5.9	96
Harvest Tomato & Herbs	1.8	94
Hearty Beef	1.3	57
Lambshank Broth	9.0	140
Minestrone	1.1	61
Pea & Ham	2.9	126
Rich Beef & Bean	2.0	76
Spring Vegetable	1.5	54
Tomato / and salt reduced	0.4	69
Vegetable	0.7	77
Vegetable & Beef	2.0	65

SOUPS - PACKET & CANNED

SAN REMO	**FAT(g)**	**CALS**
5 Minute Sachet Soups, made as directed, 250ml serve:		
Chicken Noodle, Spring Vegetable	0.3	36
Chicken Noodle salt reduced	0.4	40
Chicken & Vegetable	0.7	50
Creme of Chicken	0.9	43
Creme of Vegetable	1.0	50
Dutch Curry	0.5	49
French Onion	0.3	25
French Onion salt reduced	0.3	39
Mushroom	1.3	42
Onion	1.0	41
Onion salt reduced	1.3	46
Pea & Ham	0.8	58
Savoury Chicken Supreme	1.0	41
Tomato	1.2	56
Oodles of Noodles, made as directed, 200ml serve:		
Beef	6.8	165
Chicken	6.6	164
Cream of Chicken	8.0	174
Spring Vegetable	6.2	141
Tomato	6.4	164
Soup for a Cup, made as directed, 200ml serve:		
Chicken Noodle / and salt reduced	2.6	62
Chicken & Vegetable	1.0	50
Cream of Chicken	1.8	70
Cream of Mushroom	1.0	50
Hearty Beef	0.8	50
Pumpkin	0.8	58
Pea & Ham	1.5	70
Savoury Vegetable	0.8	58
Tomato	1.0	77
Soupremo Slimmer, made as directed, 200ml serve:		
Chicken Noodle	2.6	60
Chicken Supreme with Croutons	1.5	37
Garden Vegetable	0.3	24
Tomato & Herb	0.3	38
Soupremo with Croutons, made as directed, 200ml serve:		
Beef & Vegetables	2.8	82
Chicken	3.8	95
Chicken & Corn	3.4	96
Creamed Vegetables	4.5	110
Savoury Tomato	2.2	106

SOUPS - PACKET & CANNED

STOCKMEYER	FAT(g)	CALS
1/3 can, 265g (795g can):		
Thick Lentil Soup	7.5	222
Thick Pea Soup	5.9	215
WEIGHT WATCHERS		
Condensed Soups, ½ can, made as directed, 220g, (220g can):		
Chicken	1.1	51
Minestrone	0.2	51
Pumpkin	0.2	51
Tomato	0.2	51
Vegetable	0.4	46
Instant Soups, 1 sachet, made as directed, 200ml:		
Broccoli & Asparagus	0.8	34
Chicken with Croutons	1.6	40
Chicken Noodle, Curried Pumpkin	1.2	38
French Onion with Croutons	1.0	36
Zesty Tomato	0.2	32
WHITE WINGS		
Country Cup, made as directed, 200ml serve:		
Cream of Chicken & Corn	4.4	120
Cream of Garden Vegetable	2.2	90
Cream of Tomato with Croutons	1.7	90
Noodles Beef	0.4	106
Noodles Chicken & Corn	0.8	109
Noodles Tomato	0.8	109
Noodles Mild Curry	1.0	108
Trim Soup, 1 sachet, made as directed, 200ml:		
Chicken, Chicken & Broccoli	0.9	45
Chicken & Croutons	1.9	44
Chicken Noodle	2.0	49
Mild Chicken Curry	0.5	38
Pumpkin	0.4	43
Tomato	0.4	43
Pea & Ham	1.0	45
Vegetable	1.3	48

STOCK, FLAVOURINGS, GRAVY, HERBS & SPICES

Most stocks, flavourings, herbs & spices have only a negligible amount of fat in them and they provide an excellent way to add flavour to many dishes.

	FAT(g)	CALS
Bonox, 1 tsp., 5g	<0.1	6
Bovril, 1 tsp., 5g	<0.1	9
Chilli/Curry Powder, 1 tsp., 2.5g	0.2	8
Gravy: packet mixes, average all types, made up ¼ cup	<0.1	18
low joule packet mixes, made up ¼ cup	<0.1	10
homemade (depends on the amount of fat used in the pan), average ¼ cup	4.5	60
Herbs & Spices, 1 tsp., approx. 2g		
Allspice, Basil, Bay Leaves, Black-Pepper, Chives, Cinnamon, Dill Weed, Garlic (all types), Ginger, Lamb Seasoning, Lemon & Pepper, Marjoram, Meat Seasoning, Microwave All Purpose, Mint Leaves, Mixed Spice, Onion Salt, Onion Powder, Oregano, Parsley Flakes, Popcorn Salt, Season-All, Seasoning (Chicken, Peppercorn), Seasoned Pepper, Steak Spice, Tarragon, Thyme, Turmeric, Vanillin Sugar, White Pepper.......	<0.1	7
Cajun Seasoning, Celery Salt, Cloves, Garlic Stir Fry, Mixed Herbs, Season All (less salt), Thai Seasoning...	0.1	7
Chinese 5 spice Curry Powder, Paprika, Rosemary, Sage..	0.2	8
Coriander, Cumin, Cayenne Pepper, Salad Supreme......	0.3	9
Garlic Bread Seasoning (McCormicks)......	1.3	14
Sesame Seed (McCormicks)......	0.8	13
Mustard Powder, 1 Tbsp., 10g	2.8	46
Salt & Pepper, ¼ tsp., 1g	0.0	2
Stock, Campbell's All Natural Stock:		
375g carton: - Beef	0.4	45
- Chicken	0.8	79
- Fish	0.2	13
- Vegetable	2.6	5
Continental Stock Powder:		
Beef, 1 tsp., 5g	<0.1	12
Beef - salt reduced, 1 tsp., 5g	<0.1	15
Chicken, 1 tsp., 5g	0.1	13
Chicken - salt reduced, 1 tsp., 5g	0.1	16
Vegetable, 1 tsp., 5g	0.3	13
Stock Cubes,		
Continental: Average all flavours, each cube	0.5	10
Oxo, each cube	0.5	19

SUGAR, SWEETEENERS, SYRUPS & TOPPINGS

All of the products in this section contain little or no fat at all - however they are mostly quite high in calories.

Sugar			**FAT(g)**	**CALS**
All types of sugar, 100g serve			0.0	395

TIP *All sugars have the same fat and calorie values per 100g However, different sugars will weigh differently, ie. 1 cup of white sugar weighs approx. 230g whereas 1 cup of brown sugar may weigh between 160g & 240g depending on how firmly it is packed.*

			FAT(g)	CALS
White Sugar:	1 tsp., 4g		0.0	16
	1 Tbsp., 17g		0.0	67
	1 cup, 230g (approx.)		0.0	905
	1 sugar cube		0.0	24

Sugar includes: Dextrose, Fructose, Glucose, Lactose, Maltose, Sucrose, Brown Sugar, Castor Sugar, Coffee Sugar, Demerara, Icing Sugar, Raw Sugar.

			FAT(g)	CALS
Sweeteners:	Average all types:			
	1 sachet		0.0	4
	1 tablet		0.0	<1
	1 tsp.		0.0	2
	Splenda:	1 tsp.	0.0	2
		100g	0.0	373

Syrups & Toppings:			FAT(g)	CALS
Cane Syrup, 1 Tbsp., 25g			0.0	70
Corn Syrup, 1 Tbsp., 25g			0.0	75
Golden Syrup/Treacle,		1 tsp., 6g	0.0	19
		1 Tbsp., 25g	0.0	79
Honey, all types:	1 tsp., 6g		0.0	20
	1 Tbsp., 25g		0.0	80
Flavoured Toppings, Average all brands:				
	Caramel, 1 Tbsp., 20ml		0.2	45
	Chocolate, 1 Tbsp.		0.1	46
	Strawberry/Raspberry, 1 Tbsp.		0.0	40
Low Joule Flavoured Toppings:				
Cottee's Diet:		Caramel, 1 Tbsp.	0.2	5
		Chocolate, 1 Tbsp.	0.1	4
		Strawberry, 1 Tbsp.	0.0	3
Weight Watchers:		Apricot/Strawberry, 1 Tbsp.	0.0	4
		Chocolate, 1 Tbsp.	<0.1	6
Maple Syrup/Molasses, 1 Tbsp., 25g			0.0	63
Cottees Ice Magic, 1 Tbsp., 20g			10.0	130
Malt Extract, 1 Tbsp., 25g			0.0	75

TAKE-AWAY & FAST FOODS - GENERAL

The choices available in this area are immense. Many take-away or fast foods are high in fat and calories. However, not all fast foods can be labelled 'Junk Food'. If you are trying to limit the amount of fat in your diet try to follow these guidelines:-

* Eat small portions (eg. don't choose the biggest hamburger and the biggest serving of chips on the menu!).
* Generally speaking, bread based take-aways such as burgers, pizza, tacos etc. are more nutritious and lower in fat than their fried counterparts.
* When ordering chicken don't eat the skin.
* Ask for skim milk in your milkshake if possible.
* Avoid fried foods - they are the least nutritious and usually have the highest fat contents.
* Always eat slowly - otherwise you will still be hungry when your 'fast' food is finished.
* Remember your fat budget!

The following figures are provided as a guide only and will vary from each outlet due to cooking methods, ingredients used etc.

Chicken			**FAT(g)**	**CALS**

Deep fried pieces of chicken are high in fat - Chicken that has been rotisseried, BBQ'D, or baked is a better choice. Remember to not eat the skin!

Item			FAT(g)	CALS
Deep Fried/Fried, 1 piece, average size 100g			15.0	220
Chicken Nuggets, average size, 20g each			3.5	55
Rotisseried,	¼ small chicken:			
	breast quarter:	with skin left on	13.0	230
		without skin	7.0	180
	¼ small chicken:			
	thigh quarter:	with skin left on	19.0	275
		without skin	13.0	225
Stuffing, average serve			2.0	50
Chicken Burger, Chicken Roll			20.0	442

Chinese - Asian, *also see page 175*

Obviously this will vary greatly due to cooking methods and ingredients used. Best choices include steamed rice, vegetable or combination type dishes. Whilst sweet & sour meals are reasonably low in fat, they are often high in calories.

Item	FAT(g)	CALS
Beef Chow Mein, 250g serve	22.0	360
Beef & Black Bean Sauce, 250g serve	18.0	290
Chicken Chop Suey, 250g serve	17.0	300
Curried Prawns with Rice, 250g serve	14.0	270

TAKE-AWAY & FAST FOODS - GENERAL

Chinese - Asian, continued ...	FAT(g)	CALS
Fried Rice, 250g serve	16.0	460
Noodles, fried, 250g serve	28.8	388
Rice, steamed, 1 cup, 190g	0.5	240
Sweet & Sour Pork, 250g serve	24.0	450
Sweet & Sour Prawns, 250g serve	11.0	300
Vegetable Stir Fry/Chow Mein, 250g serve	10.0	180

Chips - Fries - Potatoes

Chips and french fries are high in fat - eat only a small serving Generally the thinner the chip or french fry, the higher the fat content.

TIP: *Potatoes roasted in their jackets are a good low fat choice - it's the filling on top of the potato that adds the fat! Go easy on the sour cream, bacon & cheese..... beans/tomato/yoghurt are a better choice as a topping.*

	FAT(g)	CALS
Chips: 1 small bucket, average size 95g	13.2	236
1 medium bucket, average size 150g	21.0	370
from a fish & chip shop, average serve 200g	28.0	495
French Fries: 1 small bucket, 80g	12.5	210
1 medium bucket, 130g	20.0	330
Potato Wedges, fried, 150g serve	18.0	340
Potato Scallops, fried, 1 only, average 100g	22.0	300
Potatoes in their Skins/Roasted, average 250g:		
with sour cream & bacon bits	19.5	355
with grilled cheese & bacon	14.0	350
with beans	0.1	215
with low fat yoghurt & bacon bits	1.5	230

Fish

Although fish itself is very low in fat, most take-away fish and fish products are deep fried and therefore high in fat and calories.

	FAT(g)	CALS
Fish, battered,crumbed deep fried, 1 piece, 150g	23.0	380
Fish & Chips, 200g chips	28.0	495
Fish Cakes, deep fried, 80g each	13.0	235
Fish Pieces/Cocktail size, deep fried, 30g each	5.0	85
Fish/Crab Sticks, deep fried, 30g each	5.0	85
Calamari Rings, 100g (8-10 rings)	9.5	205

TAKE-AWAY & FAST FOODS - GENERAL

Fried Foods/Miscellaneous		**FAT(g)**	**CALS**
Battered Saveloy, 120g each		25.0	366
Chiko Roll, 165g each		17.2	377
Dim Sims, 50g each		11.5	198
Samosa:	meat filled, 40g each	11.0	128
	vegetable filled, 40g each	10.0	128
Scallops (Potato), average 100g each		22.0	300

Greek/Lebanese, *also see pages 176 & 180*

Again, these meals will vary greatly due to cooking methods and ingredients used. Many Lebanese & Greek dishes use vegetables, lean cuts of lamb or seafood as their base. Together with the ever popular Lebanese breads, these two types of ethnic cuisine usually represent a nutritious, low fat meal.

		FAT(g)	CALS
Doner Kebab in flat lebanese bread, 300g average		20.0	560
Falafel, 30g per pattie		4.0	65
Kebabs/Souvlakia, 1 kebab		6.6	124
Moussaka, small serve, 150g		14.4	228
Spinach Pie/Spanakopita, with ricotta in filo, 1,		22.2	318
Spinach & Cheese triangles in filo:	small, 27g each	6.0	75
	large, 150g each	30.0	400
Tabbouleh, ½ cup		12.6	145

Hamburgers, ***also see Hungry Jack's & MacDonald's pages 219, 220.***

Hamburgers can be reasonably nutritious depending on the quality of meat used (fatty mince or lean mince), how much salad is included, cooking method and amount of fat used on the bun.

The main problem with hamburgers is their size. Unless you are a very active person you should choose a small hamburger. Many of the large burgers supply too much fat and too many calories for an inactive person.

Milk Bar/Take-Away Burgers, average only:	FAT(g)	CALS
Plain, 170g	17.3	384
with cheese, 195g	26.0	509
with egg, 220g	26.0	523
with bacon, 185g	24.2	472
with egg & bacon, 235g	32.0	610
with egg, bacon & cheese, 260g	40.5	730

TIP: *For homemade hamburgers you can substitute the meat pattie with a vegetarian soy protein pattie (eg.* ***Soyfeast*** *burger mix), delete any fat used in frying or on the bun, add all of the usual salad extras and have a burger that tastes just as good but has only* 3.1 350

TAKE-AWAY & FAST FOODS - GENERAL

Italian, *also see page 178* **FAT(g) CALS**

Many Italian meals are based on pasta which contains only small amounts of fat. It is the sauces that accompany the pasta that can contain all of the fat! Avoid cream or cheese based sauces - instead try to choose tomato or vegetable based ones. Also watch your serving size! Many Italian meals are rather large.

		FAT(g)	CALS
Cannelloni, average size take-away, 200g		16.8	319
Lasagne:	Meat, 220g	13.2	300
	Vegetable, 220g	8.2	220
Pizza - *see separate listing this section*			
Spaghetti/Tagliatelle/Fettuccini etc.:			
	Bolognese, 220g	10.0	330
	Carbonara (bacon & cream), 220g	23.0	400
	Marinara (seafood), 220g, no cream	8.0	320
	Napolitana (Tomato & spices), 220g	6.6	255

Mexican, *also see page 181*

Many Mexican meals are based on bread type foods such as tacos, tortillas & burritos. Main sources of fat come from the added sour cream and cheese based sauces. Opt for bean fillings - easy on the cheese. Avoid the guacomole and corn chips unless you want to spend three days of your fat budget on one meal! Otherwise, Mexican is a healthy choice.

		FAT(g)	CALS
Burrito:	bean, 1 only	11.0	310
	beef, 1 only	16.0	370
Guacamole, 1 Tbsp., 20g		4.5	42
Guacamole & Corn Chips, (1 cup 60g)		20.0	334
Nachos, with beef, beans & cheese, 1 serve		21.0	375
Taco with meat, salad & cheese, 1 only		15.0	240

Milkshakes

TIP: *A very easy way to cut down the fat in a take-away milkshake is to ask for skim milk or reduced fat milk such as Shape, Lite White etc.*

	FAT(g)	CALS
1 milkshake with whole milk, 320ml/340ml	14.0	300
1 milkshake with skim milk, 320ml/340ml	5.0	220
1 Thickshake, average all types, 300ml	10.0	275

TAKE-AWAY & FAST FOODS - GENERAL

Pies,Pasties & Sausage Rolls	**FAT(g)**	**CALS**

Not one of the better choices of take-away/fast foods due to the high fat & calorie content.

	FAT(g)	CALS
Pasties, average all brands, 170g ea	26.0	450
Pies, average all brands:		
Chicken/Chicken & Vegetable	25.0	450
Meat	26.0	435
Meat & Potato	23.0	425
Pork Pies: small (8cm diameter), 175g	46.0	650
large (12cm diameter), 435g	110.0	1600
Steak & Mushroom	22.5	400
Steak & Onion	23.0	425
Vegetable (open top pie) with cheese	17.0	380
Sausage Rolls, average all brands:		
party size, small, 40g each	8.0	122
large, 130g	22.0	378

Pizza, *also see Pizza Hut, page 221*

Pizza is a reasonably nutritious choice of take-away food which is moderately low in fat and calories. The main problem with pizza however, is that it is very easy to eat too much! Either order a small pizza or stick to one or two slices.

	FAT(g)	CALS
Average all brands, ¼ 30cm pizza (2 small slices):		
Cheese	14.0	330
Ham & Pineapple	11.0	305
Pepperoni, Cabanossi	20.0	400
Seafood	12.0	315
Supreme	14.0	350

TIP: *Generally the meat varieties of pizza contain the higher amounts of fat.*

Quiche

Quiche is generally a nutritious choice of take-away food however, if you are trying to limit the amount of fat in your diet, it is wise to only eat small portions of quiche as it does contain a high percentage of fat. Once again, great variations can occur depending on ingredients used etc.

	FAT(g)	CALS
Quiche Lorraine (Bacon/Ham & Cheese):		
average serve, 150g (small/medium wedge)	33.0	475
large piece, average 200g	44.0	633
Quiche, Spinach/Mushroom:		
average serve, 150g (small/medium wedge)	26.0	400
large piece, average 200g	35.0	530

TAKE-AWAY & FAST FOODS - GENERAL

	FAT(g)	CALS
Sandwiches *see page 186*		
Sweets/Desserts/Cakes/Pastries, *see page 38*		
Miscellaneous		
Croissants, *see Sandwiches page 186 or Breads page 28*		
Fairy Floss, 1 stick	0.0	140
Fruit Salad, average serve 200g	<0.1	115
Hot Dog, 1 only including sauce/mustard	20.5	370
Rissoles, average 170g each: Beef	15.0	330
Chicken	22.5	365
Vegetarian/Lentil	8.0	330
Roast Beef/Roast Lamb Roll	14.0	450
Spare Ribs, pork, average serve 200g	30.0	400
Toffee Apple, 1 only	0.0	155

TAKE-AWAY & FAST FOODS - POPULAR BRANDS

	FAT(g)	CALS
HUNGRY JACK'S		
Apple Pie, 80g	30.7	240
Aussie Burger, 325.5g	27.5	592
Bacon Double Cheeseburger, 175g	28.7	495
Bacon Double Cheeseburger Deluxe, 215g	36.6	570
Chicken Nuggets, 19g each: plain	4.2	59
with plum sauce, 5g	4.2	65
with sweet & sour sauce, 5g	4.2	65
French Fries, small, 76.5g	12.0	226
Grilled Chicken Burger, 179g	19.7	398
Mini Burger: plain, 113g	10.4	267
with cheese, 125.5g	14.0	311
Ocean Catch Fish Sandwich, 177g	16.3	386
Onion Rings: regular serve, 114g	22.3	397
large serve, 150g	29.3	521
Orange Juice, 227ml	0.4	84
Shakes, regular: Chocolate, 240g	7.7	277
Strawberry, 240g	7.6	282
Vanilla, 240g	7.7	279
Whopper Sandwich: plain, 286g	34.3	602
with Bacon, 303g	37.6	647
with Cheese, 298.5g	37.9	646
with Egg, 311g	35.8	632
Whopper Junior Sandwich, 153g	18.3	342
with Cheese, 165.5g	21.9	386

TAKE-AWAY & FAST FOODS - POPULAR BRANDS

K.F.C.			**FAT(g)**	**CALS**
Burgers:	Bacon & Cheese Chicken Fillet, 191g		22.3	461
	Chicken Fillet Burger, 159g		16.5	292
	Colonel Burger, 114g		14.7	286
	Works Burger, 235g		23.0	494
	Zinger Burger, 179g		17.0	423
	Bacon & Cheese Zinger, 213g		18.3	488
	Works Zinger, 247g		18.0	490
Chocolate Mousse, 75g individual serve			5.3	133
Cheesecake, 75g individual serve			7.2	176
Corn, (one cob, 156g)			2.5	180
Dinner Rolls, 21g each			1.1	60
French Fries, regular serve 117g			20.0	329
Fried Chicken, average each piece (77g edible)			14.5	207
Gravy, ¼ tub			2.1	35
Kentucky Nuggets:	18g each		2.8	47
	6 pack with sauce		16.6	300
Potato Wedges, regular serve, 152g			18.8	336
Potato mashed with gravy, small tub, 119g			1.8	80
Salads:	Bean Salad	- small, 124g	3.1	176
		- large, 500g	12.5	709
	Coleslaw	- small, 116g	6.8	129
		- large, 500g	29.5	556
	Potato	- small, 110g	6.4	108
		- large, 500g	29.0	590
Stuffing, ¼ tub, 28g			2.1	50
Tender Roast Chicken, ¼ chicken, 150g			15.9	292
McDONALDS				
Breakfast Items:	Bacon & Egg McMuffin, 142g		20.4	356
	Big Breakfast, 246g		33.9	616
	English Muffin, 68g		6.4	192
	with jam		6.4	230
	Hashbrowns, 58g		12.6	181
	Hotcakes with Maple Syrup, 252g		11.8	514
	Sausage McMuffin, 116g		18.7	338
	Sausage McMuffin with Egg, 162g		23.9	423
	Scrambled Egg McMuffin, 160g		20.6	364
Burgers:	Big Mac, 215g		26.9	503
	Cheese Burger, 117g		16.0	323
	Filet'O'Fish, 152g		16.7	384
	Junior Burger, 103g		11.4	280
	McFeast, 238g		30.9	535
	Quarter Pounder with Cheese, 205g		35.7	597

TAKE-AWAY & FAST FOODS - POPULAR BRANDS

MCDONALDS, continued...			FAT(g)	CALS
Dessert Items:	Apple Pie, 87g		17.5	275
	Apple/Oatbran Muffins, 75g		2.1	196
	McDonaldland Cookies, 60g		12.5	291
French Fries:	Small, 81g		12.6	205
	Medium, 130g		20.2	329
	Large, 169g		26.3	427
McNuggets:	19g each		3.5	54
	6 pack, 114g		20.7	325
	Sauces, per 32g serve:	B.B.Q.	0.3	51
		Mild Curry	0.2	44
		Sweet & Sour	0.5	56
		Sweet Mustard	3.3	56
Salads:	Chef Salad, 213g		7.9	112
	Garden Salad, 268g		14.5	216
	McSalad Roll, 180g		2.6	234
Salad Dressings, 1 sachet:		French (Lite)	0.0	1
		Italian	1.0	20
		Thousand Island	9.0	100
Shakes:	Chocolate:	regular, 304g	10.6	337
		large, 418g	14.6	464
	Strawberry:	regular, 304g	11.2	360
		large, 418g	15.4	495
	Vanilla:	regular, 304g	10.9	316
		large, 418g	15.0	435
Sundaes:	Average all flavours, 163g		8.0	260

PIZZA HUT, 1 slice, 1/8 medium size pizza			
Pan Pizza:	Cheese	10.4	261
	Hawaiian	10.6	293
	Supreme	16.2	343
	Super Supreme	15.0	340
Thin'N'Crispy Pizza:	Cheese	9.1	217
	Hawaiian	9.6	243
	Supreme	12.7	286
	Super Supreme	13.9	291

RED ROOSTER			
Bar-B-Q Chicken, average only, ¼ chicken:	no skin	8.0	190
	with skin	14.0	250
Spicy Skin Free:	Breast/Centre breast, 115g	5.0	175
	Breast/Side Breast, 115g	3.0	115
	Drumstick, 75g	3.3	115
	Thigh, 125g	8.3	165
	Wing, 75g	2.7	115

VEGETABLES

Like fruit, most vegetables have little or no fat and should make up a large part of your everyday diet. For many years people on 'diets' have avoided the humble potato believing it was fattening. Like bread, it is not the potato that is fattening, but what you serve with it or how you prepare it!

VEGETABLES - FRESH	**FAT(g)**	**CALS**

Where possible the weights given for the following vegetables are nett weights (ie. that portion that can be eaten)

	FAT(g)	CALS
Alfalfa Sprouts, ½ punnet 60g	<0.1	23
Ah Choi, see Bean Sprouts		
Alligator Pear, see Avocado		
Artichoke globe, 1 medium, 120g edible	0.2	25
Jerusalem, 1 small, 100g, boiled	0.1	25
Asparagus, 4 thin, 3 medium spears, 60g	<0.1	11
Asparagus Bean see Beans, Snake		
Aubergine, see Eggplant		
Australian Spinach, see Silverbeet		
Avocado: cocktail size, 20g each	4.5	40
½ small avocado, 80g (no seed)	18.0	171
½ medium, 120g (no seed)	27.0	267
100g flesh	22.6	214
Baak Choi, see Cabbage (Chinese White)		
Baby Marrow, see Zucchini		
Balsam Pear, see Melon/bitter		
Bambia, see Okra		
Bamboo Shoots, raw 1 cup	0.0	15
Bean Sprouts (Ah Choi, Nga Choi), 1 cup, 90g	0.1	19
Beans, *also see Beans/Legumes page 228*		
Broad; ½ cup boiled, 80g	0.4	35
Butter, ½ cup boiled, 70g	0.1	13
Green/French/Runner, ½ cup boiled, 70g	0.1	11
Haricot, boiled, 100g	0.7	90
Kidney, ½ cup boiled, 95g	0.4	109
Purple, ½ cup boiled, 70g	0.2	20
Snake, ½ cup boiled 70g	0.2	15
Beetroot: 1 medium, boiled & peeled, 100g	0.1	42
1 baby beet, 40g	<0.1	17
Bell Pepper, see Capsicum		
Brionne, see Choko		
Broccoli, cooked, 100g	0.3	24
Brussels Sprouts, cooked, 100g (approx. 5 sprouts)	0.3	24
Cabbage, average all varieties: ½ cup raw/shredded, 43g	0.1	5
1 cup boiled, 68g	0.1	10

VEGETABLES

VEGETABLES - FRESH

		FAT(g)	CALS
Cabbage Turnip, see Kohlrabi			
Capsicum:	Green, 1 small, 100g raw	0.1	16
	½ cup chopped, 60g	<0.1	10
	Red, 1 small, 100g raw	0.2	26
	½ cup chopped, 60g	0.1	15
Carrots:	100g raw/boiled	0.1	24
	½ cup sliced, 70g	0.1	17
Cassava, peeled, raw/boiled, 100g		0.3	134
Cauliflower,	100g boiled	0.2	19
	1 floweret raw	0.1	9
Celeriac, 100g raw/boiled		0.2	30
Celery,	1 stick raw, 20g	0.0	2
	½ cup cooked, 63g	0.1	8
Celery Knob, Celery Root, see Celeriac			
Chard /Swiss Chard, raw/boiled, 100g		0.1	22
Chayote, see Choko,			
Chicory, ½ cup raw/boiled, 80g		0.2	11
Chili peppers:	Banana, 80g each	0.2	12
	Long thin, 80g each	0.3	20
	Small green/red, 20g each	<0.1	5
Chinese Pea, see Pea, Snow			
Chives, 2 Tbsp. chopped, 8g		0.0	2
Choi Sum, see Cabbage			
Choko (Brionne, Chayote, Custard Marrow, Pepinella, Vegetable Pear), ½ cup boiled/chopped, 70g		0.2	14
Coleslaw:	home made, 100g	5.4	120
	home made with low fat dressing, 100g	2.0	90
	take-away, 100g	4.0	94
Corn, see Sweetcorn			
Courgette, see Zucchini			
Cucumber:	Incl. Apple, Common Green, Lebanese, Telegraph, Continental & Burpless, Average all types, 100g	0.1	10
Custard Marrow, see Choko			
Dasheen, see Taro			
Dong Gwa, see Gourd, Wax			
Dow Gok, see Bean, Snake			
Eggplant (Aubergine):	½ cup boiled/sliced, 100g	0.3	19
	1 slice fried in oil, 30g	7.0	70
Een Choi, see Spinach, Chinese			
Egg Fruit, see Eggplant			

VEGETABLES

VEGETABLES - FRESH	FAT(g)	CALS
Endive (Curly, Belgian), ½ cup raw/chopped, 28g	0.1	3
English Spinach, see Spinach		
Fajoli, Fava Bean, see Beans, Broad		
Fennel, ¼ cup raw/sliced, 30g	<0.1	6
¼ bulb steamed, 75g	<0.1	15
Finocchio, see Fennel		
Foo Gwa, see Melon, bitter		
Gaai Choi, see Cabbage		
Garlic: 1 clove raw, 3g	0.0	1
1 bulb roasted, 50g	1.5	50
Gau Choi, see Chives		
Gherkin, 1 pickled, 25g	<0.1	5
Ginger, 1 tsp. raw/grated or sliced	0.0	1
Girasole, see Artichoke		
Gourd: bottle, ridge, 75g	<0.1	12
wax, 75g	0.0	4
Green Pepper, see Capsicum		
Guinea Squash, see Eggplant		
Gumbo, see Okra		
Holon Dow, see Peas		
Horseradish, 1 tsp., raw	0.0	4
Italian Squash, see Zucchini		
Kale: ½ cup raw/shredded, 35g	0.3	16
½ cup cooked, 65g	0.5	12
Kau Tsoi, see Chives		
Kohlrabi (cabbage turnip), ½ cup boiled, 85g	<0.1	31
Lady's Finger, see Okra		
Leek, ½ cup raw/boiled, 50g	0.2	13
Lettuce, average all types, 2 leaves	0.0	3
Long Okra, Loofah Gourd, see Luffa, Angled		
Lotus Root, ½ root, 50-60g	<0.1	25
Luffa, Angled, 100g	0.1	12
Maize, see Sweetcorn		
Mango Squash, see Choko		
Manioc, see Cassava		
Marrow, ½ cup boiled/chopped, 110g	0.1	21
Melon, Bitter (Balsam pear or Foo Gwa), raw 100g	0.0	5
hairy, raw, 100g	0.0	11
Mirliton, see Choko		
Mixed Vegetables, frozen, ½ cup boiled, 75g	0.2	25
Mung Bean Sprouts, 1 cup, 90g	<0.1	18

VEGETABLES

VEGETABLES - FRESH	FAT(g)	CALS
Mushrooms: Button, 6, 50g approx.	0.1	12
Common, 1 large, 50g	0.1	12
Oyster, 2, 50g	0.1	17
½ cup sliced, 40g	<0.1	9
Mustard Greens, see Chives		
Neeps, see Swede		
Nga Choi, see Bean Sprouts		
Okra, cooked, 5 pods, 50g	0.1	11
Olives: Green, 1 medium, 6g	0.2	2
Black, 1 medium, 6g	1.0	8
Stuffed, 6 medium, 50g	4.3	45
Ong Choi, see Spinach		
Onions: 1 onion brown/white, average, 120g	0.1	32
½ cup, diced, raw, 55g	<0.1	13
½ cup diced, fried, 100g	5.5	160
Pickled: cocktail size, 1, 10g	0.0	3
medium size, 20g	0.0	7
Spring Onion, each	0.0	4
Onion Rings, battered or breaded, deep fried, 6 rings, 50g	13.3	200
Parsley, fresh, ¼ cup chopped, 15g	<0.1	3
Parsnip, ½ cup chopped/boiled, 75g	0.1	38
Peas: common green, fresh, raw, podded, 100g	0.4	60
common green, ½ cup boiled, 80g	0.3	40
Snow Peas/Sugar Peas, raw/boiled, 100g	0.2	35
Split Peas, green or yellow: dry 100g	2.0	300
½ cup cooked	0.7	100
Peking Cabbage, see Cabbage		
Pepinella, see Choko		
Potatoes, (average all types)		
Baked/Roast in Jacket (no fat used):		
1 medium sized potato, 150g	0.2	100
with the following toppings:		
Sour Cream, 1 Tbsp., 20g	7.7	170
Grated Cheese, 1 Tbsp., 10g	3.5	140
Grilled Bacon, ½ rasher, lean	2.2	135
Grilled Bacon, ½ rasher & 1 Tbsp. grated cheese, 10g	5.7	175

N.B. Take-away baked/roast potatoes in their jackets are often larger than 150g. See page 215.

VEGETABLES

VEGETABLES - FRESH	FAT(g)	CALS
Potatoes continued...		
Baked/roast pieces in fat, 100g piece	2.0	100
Boiled Peeled/Unpeeled, 100g	0.1	66
1 medium size, 150g	0.2	100
New Potatoes, boiled, 3 small, 90g	<0.1	60

CHIPS: The thinner cut the chip is the more fat it will absorb after deep frying. So if you are making chips at home, cut them thick.

***TIP**: Try making your own hot chips without any fat!*
As follows: Cut potatoes: into chips - precook in the microwave for 3-4 minutes. Meanwhile, mix together 1 egg white and cup of water. Remove chips from microwave and dip in egg white & water mixture.
In a plastic bag shake some Cajun Seasoning mix (or Salt & Vinegar seasoning etc.) and place chips into this bag. Shake until all chips are coated with seasoning
Place chips on an oven tray that has been sprayed with vegetable oil (eg:Pure & Simple) and bake in a hot oven for 20 minutes or until crispy.

	FAT(g)	CALS
Homemade, deep fried in oil, 100g		
Thinly cut (less than 1 cm. wide)	20.0	330
Thickly cut (1 cm. or wider)	14.0	240
Take-Away: 1 small bucket, 95g	13.2	236
1 medium bucket, 150g	21.0	370
French Fries, 100g serve	15.6	265
Oven Fried, see Vegetables Frozen		
Hash Browns, homemade, ½ cup, 90g	11.0	240
MacDonald's, 58g	12.6	181
Mashed, ½ cup, 125g:		
with whole milk & butter, average	3.5	95
with skim milk, no butter, average	0.1	75
Potato Salad, homemade with mayonnaise, 100g	10.0	220
Pumpkin: Butternut, boiled, 100g	0.7	47
Common/Queensland Blue, boiled, 100g	0.3	50
Roasted with fat, 1 piece, 100g	4.0	98
Nugget, boiled 100g	0.3	30
Purslane, ½ cup, 23g	0.0	4
Quingumbo, see Okra		
Radish: red, 1 medium, 20g	0.0	2
white, 1 medium, 20g	<0.1	3

VEGETABLES

VEGETABLES - FRESH	FAT(g)	CALS
Red Pepper, see Capsicum		
Rutabaga, see Swede		
Sai Dau, see Bean Sprouts		
Sai Yeung Choi, see Watercress		
Salsify Black (Scorzonera), ½ cup sliced, boiled, 70g	<0.1	18
Seakale, see Silverbeet		
Shallots, raw/boiled, 3, 20g	<0.1	5
Silic Gourd, Silk Gourd, see Luffa, Angled		
Silverbeet, ½ cup chopped/boiled, 60g	0.1	9
Snow Peas, 100g raw/boiled	0.2	35
Soy Bean Sprouts, ½ cup, 30g	0.8	31
Soy Beans, ½ cup, cooked, 100g	3.0	83
Spinach, average all types, raw/boiled, 100g	0.2	23
Spring Onions, 4, 50g	<0.1	13
Sprouts, see Alfalfa, Mung, Soy Bean		
Squash: average all types, 100g raw/boiled	0.2	105
Button squash, 1 medium, 35g boiled	0.1	9
Scallopini, 1 medium, 75g boiled	0.2	16
String Bean, see Beans		
Summer Squash, see Zucchini		
Sunchoke, see Artichoke, Jerusalem		
Swede, ½ cup chopped/boiled, 75g	0.0	15
Sweetcorn, 1 cob, approx. 150g (no husk)	1.4	100
Sweet Potato, average all varieties: boiled, 100g	0.1	73
baked, 100g	4.5	120
Swiss Chard, see Silverbeet		
Sze Gwa, see Luffa, Angled		
Tapioca, see Cassava		
Taro, peeled, boiled, 100g	0.2	107
Tofu (Soybean Curd): steamed, 100g	4.0	75
dried (Fu Juk), 100g	16.0	385
Tomatoes: Cherry, 5, 75g	0.1	9
Common, raw, 1 small, 100g	0.1	13
1 medium, 160g	0.1	21
1 large, 220g	0.2	29
Egg Shaped, 1 medium, 75g	<0.1	10
Tamarillo, 1 medium, 90g	<0.1	24
Tangelo, 1 medium, 130g	<0.1	48

Tomato paste, sauce, purée, *see Sauces, page 191*
Tomatoes, canned, *see Vegetables/canned, page 230*

VEGETABLES

VEGETABLES - FRESH	FAT(g)	CALS
Tseet Gwa, see Melon, Hairy		
Turnip, ½ cup boiled/chopped, 120g	0.0	25
Turnip Rooted Cabbage, see Kohlrabi		
Turnip Rooted Celery, see Celeriac		
Waterchestnuts, 1, 8g	0.1	5
Watercress, ¼ cup chopped, 8g	0.0	2
Wintermelon, see Gourd, Wax		
Winter Squash, see Pumpkin		
Witloof, see Chicory		
Windsor Bean, see Beans, Broad		
Wong Baak, see Cabbage		
Yam, ½ cup steamed, 65g	<0.3	76
Yellow Pepper, see Capsicum		
Zucchini, average all types:		
½ cup boiled/chopped, 78g	0.2	13
1 medium, boiled, 120g	0.4	18
VEGETABLE JUICE		
Tomato Juice, 200ml glass	0.0	38
V8 Vegetable Juice, 200ml glass	0.1	42
LEGUMES & BEANS - fresh, canned, dried		
Alfalfa Sprouts, 30g	0.0	12
Baked Beans in Tomato Sauce, ½ cup, 140g	0.7	95
***TIP**: Baked Beans make a great snack meal - they are very low in fat and very nutritious. Eat Up!*		
Bean Sprouts, 30g	0.0	7
Beans'n'Corn, canned, 100g	1.0	107
Blackeye Beans, Boiled, 12 cup, 95g	0.4	90
Canned, 100g	0.4	110
Dry, ½ cup, 100g	1.0	315
Blackgram Beans: boiled, 30g	0.1	27
dry, 30g	0.5	84
Borlotti Beans, canned, 100g	0.4	112
Broad Beans, boiled/steamed, 30g	0.2	12
Butter Beans, boiled, 30g	<0.1	6
Cannellini: canned, 100g	0.6	74
dry, 30g	0.4	90
Carob Bean flour, powder, 1 Tbsp., 10g	<0.1	18
Chick Peas, Garbanzo Beans: Boiled, 100g	2.3	123
Canned, 100g	1.7	103
Dry, 100g	5.3	323

VEGETABLES

LEGUMES & BEANS - fresh, canned, dried			FAT(g)	CALS
French Beans, raw or boiled, 100g			0.1	19
Haricot:	Boiled, 100g		0.7	90
	Dry, 100g		2.3	253
Heinz Beans Plus: canned bean mixes, 100g:				
	Boston Style		0.5	140
	Italian Style		1.1	103
	Mexican Style		1.3	107
	Spanish Style		0.4	98
Kidney:	Boiled, 100g		0.4	115
	Canned, 100g		0.6	87
Lentils:	Boiled, 100g		0.3	70
	Dry, 100g		2.0	261
Lima:	Boiled, 100g		0.3	71
	Canned, 100g		0.3	80
	Dry, 100g		1.7	263
Masterfoods, canned bean mixes, 100g:				
	Beans'n'Corn		0.4	97
	Chick Peas		0.8	134
	Mexican Chilli Beans		0.2	82
	Mixed Beans		0.3	54
	Red Kidney Beans		0.1	125
	Soy Beans		0.4	95
	Three Bean Mix		0.2	115
Mexican Chilli Beans, 100g			0.5	83
Mixed Beans, average all types & brands, 100g			0.4	87
Mung Beans:	Boiled, 100g		0.1	47
	Dry, 100g		1.2	283
	Sprouts, 30g		0.0	-6
Pinto, Navy & Red Beans:		Boiled, 100g	2.3	123
		Canned, 100g	1.7	103
		Dry, 100g	5.3	323
Purple Beans, boiled 100g			0.1	30
Runner Beans, raw or boiled, 100g			0.1	19
Snake Beans, raw or boiled, 100g			0.3	22
Soybeans:	Boiled, 100g		7.7	129
	Canned, 100g		5.5	92
	Dry, 100g		20.2	341

VEGETABLES

LEGUMES & BEANS - fresh, canned, dried			FAT(g)	CALS
Soybean Foods				
Soy Cheese, 30g			8.0	93
Soy Lecithin, 1 Tbsp., 20ml			12.5	122
Soy Milk, 250ml			8.0	165
also see Milk, page 166				
Miso, Soy Bean Paste, 1 Tbsp., 20g			1.0	41
Tempeh (cultured soybeans), average all brands:				
	100g uncooked		6.5	150
	100g fried		10.5	190
Tofu (Soybean Curd):	100g uncooked		5.0	90
	100g steamed, (approx. 80g raw)		4.0	75
	100g fried		9.0	140
Tofu Burgers, average 75g each:		(not fried)	5.7	134
		fried	9.7	184
Tofu Ice Cream, average all brands:				
	Regular, 1 level scoop, 50g		5.0	75
	Low Fat, 1 level scoop		1.0	60
	Soft Serve, 110g serve		8.0	158
also see Ice Cream/Tofu, page 121				
Split Peas:	Boiled, 30g		0.1	18
	Dry, 30g		0.6	89

VEGETABLES - CANNED *also see SALADS/TINNED page 183*

Average all Brands, 100g drained		FAT(g)	CALS
Artichoke, 1 heart, 50g		0.0	9
Asparagus, cuts & spears, 100g		0.1	24
Bamboo Shoots, 100g		<0.1	15
Beans:	Baked Beans	0.4	104
	Broad Beans	0.2	50
	Butter Beans	0.5	94
	Four Bean Mix	0.6	97
	Golden Butter Beans	0.1	16
	Green Beans	0.1	16
	Kidney Beans	0.5	95
	Soybeans	5.6	94
Beetroot, Baby beets, slices		0.1	45
Carrots, Baby, Julienne		0.1	16
Chick Peas (Garbanzo Beans)		1.0	121
Corn Kernels		0.7	98
Corn, Creamed		0.7	81

VEGETABLES

VEGETABLES - CANNED		FAT(g)	CALS
Corn, Lima & Capsicum		0.4	99
Cucumber		<0.1	76
Diced Capsicum		0.1	21
Lotus Root		<0.1	20
Mixed Vegetables, average:		0.4	34
Mushrooms:	in Butter Sauce	1.0	28
	Champignons in Brine	0.4	16
Peas, green		0.4	60
Peas & Carrots,		0.3	41
Potatoes, eg. Tiny Taters (**Edgell**)		0.1	51
Red Cabbage		0.2	25
Sauerkraut		0.2	13
Tomatoes, all types		0.2	20
Water Chestnuts		1.0	40

VEGETABLES - FROZEN
Average all brands, 100g

Item		FAT(g)	CALS
Beans, Baby, Green, Golden		0.1	34
Broad Beans		0.5	58
Broccoli		0.3	23
Brussel Sprouts		0.3	30
Carrots, all types		0.2	22
Cauliflower		0.1	17
Cauliflower in White Sauce (**McCain**)		1.8	44
Corn Kernels:	100g	0.9	93
	Cobs, per 100g	0.6	65
Logan Farm, Corn Nuggets:			
	1 oven heated	1.3	32
	1 deep fried	6.3	76
Edgell-Birdseye, 100g			
	Broccoli in Cream Sauce with Almonds	2.5	46
	Cauliflower in Cheese Sauce	2.3	50
	'Green Dragon' Cantonese	0.4	58
	'Green Dragon' Chow Mein	0.4	31
	'Green Dragon' Sweet'n'Sour	0.3	31
	Vegetables in Cheese Sauce	3.6	87
	Vegetables in Herb Sauce	0.1	30
Mixed Vegetables:	Beans/Carrot/Corn	0.5	46
	Carrot/Cauliflower/Broccoli	0.2	26
	Peas/Beans/Corn	1.0	61
	Peas/Carrot/Cauliflower	0.3	35
	Peas/Corn/Capsicum	0.7	70

VEGETABLES

VEGETABLES - FROZEN	FAT(g)	CALS
Onions, chopped, 100g	0.3	25
Peas, all types, 100g	0.4	50
Spinach, 100g	0.3	20

POTATO CHIPS - POTATO PRODUCTS - OVEN FRIES - FROZEN

N.B. The figures given for the following products are for 100g of frozen/uncooked product. You must add extra for any fat used in cooking.

	FAT(g)	CALS
On average, for every 100g of chips that are deep fried in oil you will need to ADD:................... to the amount for the uncooked chips.	5.0	44

If you dry bake the frozen chips in your oven then you do not need to add anything to the figures listed below.

(Remember, 100g of chips is only a small serving!)

BIRD'S EYE 100g frozen, uncooked		FAT(g)	CALS
Chips:	Canola Oven Fries	4.0	147
	Chunky	4.0	141
	Crinkle Cut 5mm	7.0	171
	Crinkle Cut 10mm	4.0	144
	French Fries	6.2	182
	Hot & Spicy / Extra Hot & Spicy	5.0	153
	Multifries	4.2	149
	Straight Cut	3.8	125
Hash Browns		7.0	171
Potato Gems, all flavours, 100g		9.2	158
Potatoes in Cheese Sauce, 100g		5.0	116

FARMLAND 100g frozen/uncooked		FAT(g)	CALS
Oven Fries:	Crinkle Cut	4.2	140
	Straight Cut	4.0	140

FINDUS	FAT(g)	CALS
Pommes Noisettes, 30g (6 pieces)	2.5	57

VEGETABLES

POTATO CHIPS - POTATO PRODUCTS - OVEN FRIES FROZEN

McCAIN 100g frozen, uncooked		**FAT(g)**	**CALS**
Healthy Choice, Country/Straight Cut		3.0	131
Potato Cakes, 100g		12.6	324
Potato Patties, 100g		9.9	189
Super Crisps		13.1	256
Superfries:	Crinkle Cut	4.4	155
	Chunky Cut	4.1	137
	Polyunsaturated Crinkle Cut	5.8	194
	Polyunsaturated Straight Cut	4.6	194
	Shoestring	6.8	172
Super Spirals		9.0	196
Taterbites, 100g		8.9	192
SARA LEE frozen, uncooked			
Tasmanian Salmon Fans, 33g each		2.7	53
Viennese Fans, 33g each		2.6	57
Viennese Rosti:	Cheese, 33g each	3.0	65
	Plain, 33g each	3.1	62
	Pumpkin, 27g each	3.0	51

VEGETABLES - DRIED, DEHYDRATED

Average all brands			
Instant Mashed Potato, plain/onion, 20g dry powder only		2.2	95
Onion, dehydrated flakes, 100g flakes		0.0	57
Sun Dried Tomatoes (not in OIL!), 30g		<0.1	85
packed in oil, 30g		5.0	120
Vegetables & Noodles (**Dewcrisp**), 100g dry		<0.1	77
Continental Surprise vegetables, 100g dry:			
Peas		0.2	85
Peas Minted		0.2	94
Peas & Carrots		0.1	94
Peas & Corn		0.3	94
Green Beans		0.2	71
Continental Deb:	Plain, 118g pkt., dry	11.4	477
	20g serve, dry	1.9	81
	With Onion, 118g pkt., dry	10.8	474
	20g serve, dry	1.8	80

YOGHURT

Choose low fat or reduced fat yoghurts and enjoy them as healthy snacks, or use low fat yoghurt as an alternative to milk, sour cream or cream in many meals, eg. home-made muffins, salad dressings, potato toppings etc.

ALL BRANDS & VARIETIES	FAT(g)	CALS
200g serve, average		
Natural	7.0	165
Natural, low fat, with sugar	0.3	160
Natural, low fat, no sugar	0.3	105
Fruit flavours	4.5	190
Fruit flavours, low fat, with sugar	0.2	185
Fruit flavours, low fat, no sugar	0.2	95
VARIOUS BRANDS:		
ATTIKI 200g carton or serve		
Acidophilus: Apricot	0.2	110
Honey	0.2	128
Natural	0.2	86
Strawberry	0.2	112
Country Style	6.8	196
Reduced Fat: Apricot/Fruit Salad	3.0	172
Cherry/Strawberry	3.0	170
Honey	3.0	184
Natural	3.0	157
BORNHOFFEN 200g carton or serve		
Acidophilus: Fruit flavours	5.8	206
Natural	7.2	168
BROWNE'S 200g carton or serve		
Diet: Appleberry/Melon Basket	0.3	102
Cherry Banana	0.2	116
Dessert Yoghurt: Cherry & Coconut	6.6	168
Creamy Vanilla	6.8	223
Hazelnut Toffee	7.6	255
Encore: *see Dairy Desserts page 44*		
Low Fat: Apple & Rhubarb	0.2	177
Mandarin Orange	0.3	180
Natural	0.3	108
Peach & Plum	0.3	160
Strawberry	0.3	168
Natural	6.6	168

YOGHURT

VARIOUS BRANDS		FAT(g)	CAL
BROWNE'S 200g carton or serve continued...			
Traditional:	Apricot	5.6	234
	Muesli	6.4	238
	Strawberry	5.6	220
BULLA			
Lite'n'Healthy, Fruit Yoghurt, 200g		2.0	186
Reduced Fat, Plain Yoghurt, 200g		0.2	156
Soft Serve Yoghurt, 100g serve		5.5	142
Yohoho Drinking Yoghurt, 100g serve		0.9	89
CABOOLTURE 200g carton or serve			
Real Fruit:	Flavours	5.8	226
	Natural	7.2	168
DAIRY FARMERS 200g carton or serve			
Traditional:	Low Fat Yoghurt	0.3	99
	Natural	6.8	153
DAIRYLITE (CABOOLTURE)			
Dairylite Diet, all flavours, 200g carton or serve		0.2	86
Dairylite Lo, Fruit flavours, 200g carton or serve		0.4	150
DANONE 200g carton or serve			
Diet Lite low fat, sugar free:			
	Average all fruit flavours	0.2	95
	Vanilla	0.2	87
Full Fat Fruit Yoghurt:			
	Fruit Flavours, Fruit Salad	4.4	185
	Vanilla & Fruit flavours	4.4	192
Light & Fruity low fat:			
	Average all flavours	0.3	137
Danino 150g carton:			
	Banana/Banana & Strawberry	1.9	136
	Strawberry/Tropical/Vanilla	1.9	144
FRESH'N'FRUITY (N.Z.) 150g carton			
Average all flavours		1.0	100

YOGHURT

VARIOUS BRANDS			FAT(g)	CALS
JALNA 200g carton or serve				
	Bio Dynamic Natural		9.0	196
	Leben Natural		6.4	132
	Mild Continental Natural		6.4	136
	Premium Blend Natural		9.8	194
	Skim Milk:	Berryfruits/Tropical	0.2	172
		Honey	0.4	142
		Natural	0.2	104
		Vanilla	0.2	120
MUNCH BUNCH (Dairy Farmers), 200g carton or serve				
	Banana		2.0	182
	Chocolate		2.8	206
	Strawberry		2.0	190
	Vanilla		2.0	187
OAK 200g carton or serve				
	Fruit Yoghurt:	Apricot	4.4	184
		Fruit Salad/Mango	4.4	181
		Passionfruit/Strawberry	4.4	178
		Vanilla	6.3	208
SKI 200g carton or serve				
	Diet: no added sugar			
		Blueberry/Wild Berries	0.3	95
		Fruit Salad	0.3	96
		Strawberry	0.4	95
	D'Lite, 200g carton or serve			
		average all flavours	1.9	180
	Divine, 200g carton or serve			
		Forest & Field flavours, average	8.0	222
		Fruit Passion flavours, average	8.0	214
		Sunshine Fruits flavours, average	8.0	216
	Double Up, 200g carton:			
	Vanilla Yoghurt with:	Apple & Rhubarb	1.6	198
		Black Cherry	1.6	184
		Blueberries	1.6	184
		Fruit & Nut	9.8	292
		Muesli	5.8	272
		Pineapple & Coconut	6.8	214
		Strawberry Redcurrant	1.6	188

YOGHURT

VARIOUS BRANDS		FAT(g)	CALS
SKI 200g carton or serve continued...			
Fruit:	Apricot/Strawberry	4.4	193
	Forest Fruit/Fruit Salad	4.4	196
	Passionfruit/Raspberry	4.4	188
	Strawberry	4.5	194
Lite:	Apricot/Apricot & Vanilla	0.3	159
	Berries & Cherries	0.3	167
	Five Fruits & Vanilla	0.3	165
	Fruit Salad	0.3	162
	Mango & Peach/Raspberry	0.3	153
	Strawberry/Strawberry & Vanilla	0.4	160
WEIGHT WATCHERS 200g carton or serve			
Skim Milk:	Fruit Salad	0.3	94
	Grapefruit & Mandarin	0.4	102
	Natural	0.4	98
	Strawberry	0.4	92

YO-GO *see Dairy Desserts page 44*

YOPLAIT		FAT(g)	CALS
Fruit Yoghurt:	All flavours incl. vanilla, 100g	2.2	102
	200g carton	4.4	204
Light(low fat):	Vanilla Basket flavours, 100g	0.5	96
	200g carton	1.0	192
	Other flavours, average, 100g	0.2	84
	200g carton	0.4	168
Non-Cholest:	Average all flavours, 100g	0.1	89
	200g carton	0.2	178
Petit Miam:	Average all flavours, 100g	6.8	147
	60g carton	4.0	88
Silhouette:	Average all flavours, 100g	0.2	47
	200g carton	0.4	94
Vanilla with:	Crunchy Muesli, 100g	4.1	147
	175g carton	7.2	257
	Fruit & Nut, 100g	5.6	149
	175g carton	9.8	261
	Fruit of the Forest/Strawberry, 100g	2.5	103
	175g carton	4.4	181

YOGHURT

VARIOUS BRANDS		FAT(g)	CALS
YOPLAIT continued			
Yoplus:	Fruit - average all flavours, 100g	3.0	88
	200g carton	6.0	176
	Natural, 100g	3.5	80
	200g carton	7.0	160
YO-SPLIT 200g carton or serve			
Vanilla with:	Apricot	2.8	208
	Fruit of Paradise	2.8	214
	Muesli & Fruit	7.0	360
	Strawberry	2.8	218
YO-WHIP 175ml. carton or serve, average all flavours		5.0	160

NOTES

78c 1½. 270 Cals = 4½ PTS

NOTES

52c = 1pt.

Milk for Day,

Porridge 2

Weatabix 1½

Muesli 2 — 4.

Prunes 1p.

Cereal Bars 1½.

Fruit Juice 2-1.

Banana, 1-2.

Wine. 1"

~~Dry~~ white 1

Red 1½

Sherry 1

Liquer 1½

Liquer Coffee 3½.

Toast 105

Mince Pie 193

Prunes 3 = 52cal = 1point

140-00 -wine 2 glasses wo wo -

95-00

crumpets 90 cal.